KT-385-166

Azmina Govindji BSc RD is a consultant nutritionist and registered dietitian, broadcaster, best-selling author and Master NLP Practitioner.

She spent eight years as the National Consultant on Diet and Diabetes when she was Chief Dietitian to Diabetes UK. This experience makes her particularly qualified to write this book, as GI is a concept that has been used in diabetes for years. She runs her own practice providing dietetic consultancy to the food industry, healthcare professionals, the media, and national organisations such as the British Heart Foundation and Diabetes Research and Wellness Foundation. She is currently Chairperson of the British Dietetic Association (BDA) PR Committee.

A regular contributor to numerous magazines, she also appears on TV and radio, and is frequently quoted in the national press as spokesperson to the British Dietetic Association. She is author of 10 books, including *Healthy Eating for Diabetes* with Anthony Worrall Thompson and *Think Well to Be Well* with Nina Puddefoot.

Nina Puddefoot is a Master Practitioner and Certified NLP Trainer and development life coach. She works with leading-edge and creative models of thinking within multinational organisations and industries, as well as individuals worldwide.

She is an author and a regular presenter of public programmes, talks and workshops and regularly makes contributions to radio, newspapers and magazines, such as *The Daily Mail*, *New Woman* and *Family Circle*.

AZMINA GOVINDJI BSc RD AND NINA PUDDEFOOT

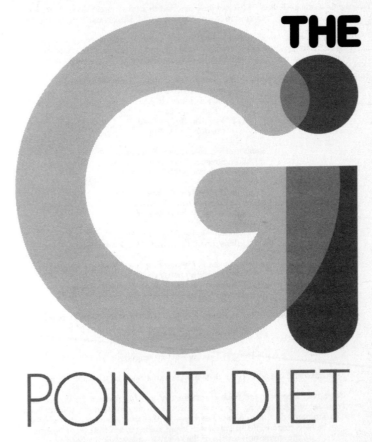

THE
Gi
POINT DIET

LOSE WEIGHT FOREVER –
WITH THE REVOLUTIONARY
POINT-COUNTING SYSTEM

Vermilion
LONDON

1 3 5 7 9 10 8 6 4 2

Text (excluding GiP values and GiP tables) © Azmina Govindji and Nina Puddefoot 2004
GiP values and GiP tables © Azmina Govindji 2004

Azmina Govindji and Nina Puddefoot have asserted their moral right to be identified as the
authors of this work in accordance with the Copyright, Design and Patents Act 1988.

All rights reserved. No part of this publication may be reproduced, stored in a retrieval
system, or transmitted in any form by means electronic, mechanical, photocopying,
recording or otherwise, without the prior permission of the copyright owner.

First published in the United Kingdom in 2004 by Vermilion,
an imprint of Ebury Press
Random House UK Ltd
Random House
20 Vauxhall Bridge Road
London SW1V 2SA

Random House Australia (Pty) Limited
20 Alfred Street, Milsons Point, Sydney
New South Wales 2061, Australia

Random House New Zealand Limited
18 Poland Road, Glenfield
Auckland 10, New Zealand

Random House (Pty) Limited
Endulini, 5A Jubilee Road, Parktown 2193, South Africa

Random House UK Limited Reg. No. 954009
www.randomhouse.co.uk
Papers used by Vermilion are natural, recyclable products
made from wood grown in sustainable forests.

A CIP catalogue record is available for this book from the British Library.

ISBN: 0091900093

Designed and typeset by seagulls

Printed and bound in Great Britain by Bookmarque Ltd, Croydon, Surrey

The advice offered in this book is not intended to be a substitute for the advice
and counsel of your personal physician. Always consult a medical practitioner before
embarking on a diet, or a course of exercise. Neither the authors nor the publisher
can be held responsible for any loss or claim arising out of the use, or misuse,
of the suggestions made, or the failure to take medical advice.

Whilst the following trademarks are mentioned in *The Gi Point Diet*, the book is not endorsed
by any of the trademark owners: Ryvita is a registered trademark of Associated British Food;
Grape-Nuts is a registered trademark of the General Mills Company; Bran Flakes, Raisin
Splitz and Sultana Bran are unregistered trademarks of the Kellogg Company; All Bran,
Special K, Cornflakes, Rice Krispies and Nutrigrain are registered trademarks of the Kellogg
Company; Quorn is a registered trademark of Marlow Foods Limited; Snickers, Twix, Mars
and M&M are all registered trademarks of Masterfoods, UK; Splenda is a registered
trademark of McNeil Nutritionals, a Division of McNeil-PPC, Inc.; Nesquik and Shredded
Wheat are registered trademarks of Nestle U.K. Limited; Hovis is a registered trademark of
RHBB (IP) Limited; Weetabix is a registered trademark of Weetabix Limited.

The authors and publishers have made all reasonable efforts to contact
copyright holders for permission, and apologise for any omissions or errors
in the form of credit given. Corrections may be made in future printings.

Dedicated to ...

As far as I can remember, this is one of the hardest projects I have ever had to do. As I look back on my mother's life, it is she who has inspired me to succeed and to be the very best that I can be. Her foresight and courage have been a living example to me. I would like to dedicate this book to my loving mum, Roshan.

Azmina

My love and thanks go to my dear mum, Joan, and my long-suffering partner, Richard, for their unconditional love and support with my writing and teachings.

Thanks to my close-knit circle of friends, too, for their support and keeping my spirits uplifted.

And, to my co-author, Az, my dear friend and business partner, without whom this book would never have happened.

Nina

Acknowledgements

We'd like to say a huge thank you to our special colleague, Smita Ganatra, whose analytical mind and dietetic expertise have contributed to the meticulous development of the point system. Various diet and exercise experts have also been part of the team: Dr Wynnie Chan, Nigel Denby, Kate Arthur, Sue Baic and Rosita Evans.

The real genius behind such a book is the original researcher. We are indebted to Dr Jenkins and his team; the authors of the GI international tables: Foster-Powell, Holt and Brand-Miller; McCance and Widdowson's *Composition of Foods*; Jill Davies and John Dickerson's *Nutrient Content of Food Portions*; as well as Dr Tony Leeds and other authors of *The New Glucose Revolution*, which was great bedtime reading! Thanks also to the host of dietitians who shaped our writing by contributing their personal views on the use of GI – they have been a great encouragement.

To our editor, Amanda Hemmings – thank you for offering us the opportunity to share our concepts and work by being able to express them in this book. And the most special of all, Azmina's husband Shamil and her young children, Shazia and Bizhan, who often stayed up till the early hours of the morning tirelessly supporting the development of the final manuscript.

To each other – as co-authors and dear chums, we

consider ourselves so fortunate to have shared this experience, always being an inspiration to one another, especially when times got tough! This is our special thank you to each other for shared patience and belief – we make a rich team and have a lot of fun along the way.

We would also especially like to thank the following people:

- **Smita Ganatra BSc RD**
  Chief dietitian, Central Middlesex Hospital
  For her professional expertise in assisting in the development of the Gi Point System.

- **Dr Wynnie Chan BSc PhD RPHNutr**
  Former Nutrition Scientist for the British Nutrition Foundation
  For providing some of the data analysis.

- **Nigel Denby BSc RD**
  Registered Dietitian, Channel 4's Fit Farm
  For his contribution in helping to make this diet more suitable for men and assisting with the scientific reviews.

- **Kate Arthur BSc RD**
  Registered Dietitian and Sports Accredited Dietitian
  For her contribution to some of the chapters.

● **Sue Baic BSc RD**

Registered Dietitian and Lecturer in Nutrition at Bristol University

For providing some of the data analysis.

● **Rosita Evans**

Qualified Fitness Instructor

For kindly permitting us to use extracts of her book, *Rosie's Armchair Exercises*, published by Discovery Books, 29 Hacketts Lane, Woking, GU22 8PP; tel: 01932 400800.

CONTENTS

EXPERT QUOTES AND TESTIMONIALS

You only need to scan the bookshelves to see the vast range of diet books out there. The hottest fad, the latest quick fix. This book, to me, makes far more sense. Firstly, it's written by experts in the field who have personal experience working with real people who need to manage their weight. Secondly, it is based on GI and calories. GI has been used in diabetes for years, and because low-GI foods can make you feel less hungry, you eat less without thinking you're 'on a diet'. Thirdly, in its application of GI to a healthy diet, it probably goes further than any other GI diet book out there and has all the makings of a well thought-out plan. And then there's the icing on the cake. Even with the most effective dietary advice, any new way of eating might be short lived unless you have prepared yourself mentally. Enjoy the strong willpower boosters and treasure chest of practical tips.

Dr Chris Steele, resident doctor on ITV's This Morning

This is a great book for all those who want to lose weight without losing their health. Nutritional science is blended with practical help to provide a safe plan for permanent weight control.

Dr Derrick Cutting, GP and author of Stop that heart attack!

The key to long-term weight management is to find a lifestyle plan that isn't restrictive and that fits with who you are. Az and Nina have, in my view, gone a long way to making this programme clear, realistic and engaging enough for both men and women. Their simple point system, guidelines and practical tips encourage you to eat the right foods without having to think too much. The book focuses on what you can do rather than what you mustn't, and addresses the importance of a healthy lifestyle, not just the importance of losing weight. The advice is practical and suitable for the whole family. I particularly like the Quick Start Guide, as I know many of my patients just want to get on with it.

Motivation, that essential ingredient to successful weight reduction, is integral to the whole programme, and the book shows you how to change your thinking to help you lose weight. The authors take you on a voyage of discovery and explain the concepts behind what they advise. A refreshing book that I'm sure will be a source of help to many people.

Dr Rob Hicks MB BS, DRCOG, MRCGP, GP, writer and broadcaster

The key to long-term weight loss is the same as it's always been – keep it slow and steady. The most successful slimming plans are based on a weight loss of 1–2 lb per week. Some quick-fix diets promise that you'll achieve your perfect figure in weeks – though they may be tempting, they don't help you in the long term and some can be potentially damaging if you miss out on key food groups. This diet is about healthy weight management – losing it slowly and steadily and taking on strategies that will help you to keep the weight off in the long term. This makes it a valuable guide for slimmers as well as people who just want to eat well.

GI cannot be used in isolation and the authors are very aware of this. They even offer the Gi Point value of some calculated mixed meals – based on the scientific formula for predicting how a meal affects blood glucose.

The authors have received some excellent support from colleagues in the opening chapter, and their advice is neatly packaged into practical tips and tools that encompass sound nutritional principles around healthy eating, physical activity, motivation and realistic calorie reduction.

Dr Wendy Doyle RD PhD, Former National Public Relations Officer to the British Dietetic Association

GI can be used in the management of diabetes as part of an overall healthy lifestyle. But using the glycaemic index of foods is cumbersome and the approach to living with diabetes needs to be simple and flexible. This is where the authors have taken the GI research and transformed it into a programme that incorporates those healthy eating and weight management guidelines without an index in sight. The simple point system allows for a measured calorie intake and encourages healthy low GI, low fat choices. I have known Azmina for many years and worked with her when she was Chief Dietitian at Diabetes UK and have always admired her professionalism and her commitment to excellent communication so that people can understand and take on the challenge of self management.

Suzanne Lucas, Director of Research and Care, Diabetes UK

This book promotes heart-healthy foods like wholegrains, pulses, nuts, fish, fruit and vegetables. Reducing the incidence of obesity by incorporating sensible guidelines can go a long way to help prevent heart problems.

As Ethnic Strategy Co-ordinator for the British Heart Foundation, I am always looking for simple ways to help ethnic groups in the UK enjoy their traditional cuisine whilst keeping to a healthy diet. The authors in this book have found a way of doing both. You'll notice that many traditional South Asian foods like Bangladeshi and basmati rice, and dahls are also low-GI foods and are encouraged within the context of a low saturated fat diet. Even the more unusual African Caribbean starchy foods like matoki, cassava and yams are included as part of the choice. Since South Asians are around 50% more likely to suffer from coronary heart disease, sensible eating and regular physical activtiy are especially important.

I have had the opportunity to work with both Azmina and Nina on the Department of Health video 'Enjoying Healthy Living' and I know they are committed, professional and have great attention to detail. I would like to congratulate them for producing such an excellent resource.

Qaim Zaidi, Ethnic Strategy Co-ordinator, British Heart Foundation

GI has come to be recognised as a vital tool in successful diabetes management but, until now, it has had its limitations. In their inimitable style, Azmina and Nina have taken GI to another level, combining the best of GI ranking with aspects of traditonal dietary thinking. While this book is not written specifically with diabetes in mind, it does offer a clear and inspiring route to sensible weight loss based on good blood glucose control, which is especially useful to people living with diabetes.

James Rogers LLB, Executive Director, Diabetes Research & Wellness Foundation

There is established scientific evidence for the value of GIs in blood glucose control and satiety. The most exciting thing about this book is that it takes this one step further by combining the GI value of food with its calorie density to give a weight management programme that is practical and embodies all the principles of healthy eating.

Smita Ganatra RD, Chief Dietitian – London

It's great to have a good sensible and accurate book on this approach written by a dietitian!

Amanda Wynne BSc RD, Registered Dietitian

Views from qualified dietitians on the Glycaemic Index

I would be happy to use any weight-reducing plan that generally followed healthy principles, which I know this book does.

Sue Baic BSc RD, Lecturer in Nutrition – Bristol University

What a fantastic idea: a book like this fills the real need for a low-GI diet plan for weight management. A book that really makes the Glycaemic Index easy to under-stand and use in everyday lives has been long awaited.

I would definitely use the GI approach when giving advice on weight management. It can be kept simple and the beauty of it is that it fits well with healthy eating advice. I really believe that low-GI eating as part of a healthy balanced diet is the way we should all be eating.

Kate Arthur BSc RD, Registered Dietitian and Sports Accredited Dietitian, London

Since insulin is the key trigger to storing glucose, as well as the sentry that keeps those fat cells intact, it is crucial to maintain low insulin levels when you are trying to lose weight. Low-GI foods are broken down at a slow, steady rate so there is the feeling of fullness for longer. I believe in the concept that a slimming plan must be balanced: 50 per cent of the plate as veg, 25 per cent as protein which are low in saturates and 25 per cent carbohydrate in the form of low-GI foods. This is embraced by the Gi Point Diet!
Baldeesh Rai BSc RD Chief Dietitian – The Natural Health Show, *Sony TV*

The GI is a great example of how the healthy eating message is being fine-tuned as nutrition knowledge evolves. Balanced low-GI eating appears to not only promote good health, but helps with weight control thanks to its effects on appetite regulation.
Lyndel Costain BSc RD, Dietitian for BBC's Diet Trials

In my work with overweight children in Bristol, we use elements of a GI approach as a way of trying to control appetite. I like the idea of it being very practical, so that it would be easy for people to plan their meals around.
Jill Scott BSc RD, Registered Dietitian, Bristol

Current evidence indicates that low-GI diets help reduce the risk of heart disease and diabetes. In practice, it seems that low-GI diets also help reduce hunger, which is an added benefit for anybody who is trying to lose weight.

Dympna Pearson SRD, Consultant Dietitian and
Freelance Trainer – Leicestershire

Using GI in a slimming plan makes a whole lot of sense. Incorporating low-GI foods as a basis for menu planning (alongside good basic balance-eating of course!) is a very good way to help the body to relearn appropriate appetite cues.

Jennette Higgs BSc SRD RPHNutr, Accredited Sports
Dietitian, Food To Fit Nutrition Consultancy –
Northamptonshire

Lower-GI foods do assist with satiety and certainly help with improved blood glucose profiles and, because they tend to be bulkier, people don't tend to eat so much or rather overeat. I think ideas for lower-GI snacks is very useful.

Jan Philpott BSc RD, Diabetes Dietitian – Moray

Within the Primary Care Service of NHS Greater Glasgow, we have developed a GI-based approach in our leaflet 'Eastern and Western food ideas' (see Further Information and Support, page 349). Our South Asian patients like this format so I have been using it for heart healthy eating as well as weight management.

Sunita Wallia BSc MSc SRD, Community Dietitian –
Glasgow

I'm a great fan of the GI. I use it with diabetics and reactive hypoglycaemic patients.

Ruth Redman BSc RD, Chief Dietitian – Guildford

Testimonials from dieters

The first thing I thought when I browsed through the book was 'I can do this. I can do this'. The GiPs tables covered so many of my usual foods and when I looked at the other dieters plans, I could see how easy it was to keep to. I spent the weekend reading through the book more thoroughly, and then I made my shopping list. Having the right foods accessible has been the key.

My best learning so far is the v,v,p,c, which I memorise as 'veggie veggie protein carbs'. I keep a picture of that plate in my mind when I go to restaurants or the sandwich bar. I chose a lasagne at the pub the other day and the menu said I could have chips or new potatoes, and veg or salad. When I thought about v,v,p,c, I could see that my pasta was the carb, beef was the protein, and I needed to choose the veg and the salad to get it right. It filled me up, it was delicious and I was keeping to the eat a rainbow guidelines at the same time. When I eat a sandwich, I use the bread as the carb, the filling as the protein, and I make sure I always have a salad (in the sandwich or as extra) as well as a fruit for the veggie bit.

Caroline

I have found it a great help. I have realised that even when I have days when I feel I have slipped a bit, I am making much better food choices without even thinking about it! I am enjoying the snacks and look forward to them without feeling guilty, especially when people at work keep asking 'Are you eating again?' I can't thank you enough for bringing me this plan because I don't feel I am going without anything and my meals and my low energy levels are a thing of the past! My skin looks so much better too.

Christine

The best thing about this diet is I don't feel hungry. Normally the minute I start a diet, it feels like I've been on it for a month already. I feel like devouring the most calorific, sugary and fatty cream cake going. Now for the first time, I don't feel like I'm on a diet. In fact, the GiP programme forces me to have a snack when I wouldn't normally have one. That's what's helped me to cut down the crisps and chocolates on my way home from work. And I'm not known for my self-discipline! I've even replaced late night TV binge-snacking with other tasty and healthier snacks.

You get used to the GiP system very quickly, and you get to know your favourite low-GiP alternatives. I now eat most things, including some I didn't before. The result? I have lost almost a stone. I look forward to my weigh-day each week, knowing that I'll have lost 1–2 lbs (and then jump up and punch the air – what a feeling!). Not only do I look better and feelgood, I know that my kids are also eating healthy food without us really having to try. I wish this book was around years ago – I'd recommend it to anyone.

Paul

FOREWORD

Obesity is a growing national problem. The latest National Diet and Nutrition survey on adults aged 19–64 found that a quarter of men are obese, and a further 42% are overweight. One in five women are obese and a further 32% are overweight. With the associated health risks, now is a crucial time for us to take notice and find an attractive yet simple strategy that is practical and achievable. On reading these pages, I think Azmina and Nina have created a programme that not only encompasses good healthy eating advice, but also offers you a balanced, simple approach to choosing your favourite foods whilst the weight sheds off slowly and steadily.

The Gi Point Diet provides a flexible, realistic and forgiving approach to dieting. It is not about avoiding foods, but simply eating what you like within healthy boundaries – and it even allows for those occasional naughty bites and moments when you really need comfort food. Inspirational and encouraging, it not only provides the motivation you need to stick to the diet, but also transforms your entire relationship with food.

The Glycaemic Index (GI) has been used in diabetes for years. The concept is not new, and the beneficial effect on blood glucose after eating low-GI foods is well documented. What's new here is the unique way that GI has been applied to help you lose weight. The authors are well aware of the limitations of using GI alone and so they have originated a system that incorporates the *good* bits of the GI approach, within the context of overall healthy eating strategies. The healthy low-GI foods that the diet recommends make a whole lot of sense. Pasta, wholegrain cereals, beans, lentils, nuts, fruit, veg, grainy bread, basmati rice – filling not fattening. The system automatically takes into account the GI and calorie density of foods, gives guidance on satisfying portion sizes, offers a wealth of practical tips on healthy eating, provides achievable fitness targets, gives snacking, shopping and eating out advice, and lots more.

Dietitians and doctors have tried for years to encourage people to choose balanced foods in limited quantities so that they can achieve a healthy weight. You just need to look around you to see that it's not working. This simple point-counting system with its dietary guidelines offers a novel, down-to-earth, achievable and sustainable programme all rolled into one. It's about eating, not guilt. It's about lifestyle change, not a quick fix. It's about success through the *right* carbs, not missing out on your favourite carbs.

The authors are very experienced in their fields. I have personally worked with Azmina, and an upbeat, practical attitude is very much her style.

Complementing her skills with the inspiring thinking of a life coach like Nina, makes for a hearty cocktail of fun and knowledge.

Dr Hilary Jones MBBS
GP and resident doctor for ITV's GMTV

Commitment

Until one is committed there is hesitancy, the chance
    to draw back,
always ineffectiveness.
Concerning all acts of initiative (and creation)
there is one elementary truth,
the ignorance of which kills countless ideas
and splendid plans:
that the moment one definitely commits oneself,
then Providence moves too.
All sorts of things occur to help one
that would otherwise never have occurred.
A whole stream of events issues from the decision,
raising in one's favour all manner
of unforeseen incidents and meetings
and material assistance,
which no man could have dreamt
would have come his way.

Goethe

YOUR INTRODUCTION TO THE Gi POINT DIET

Congratulations! By picking up this book you've made that all-important first step towards becoming the slimmer, healthier, happier 'you' that *you* want to be. *Why? Because* the Gi Point Diet *really works.*

What are the three main reasons why dieters give up with other diet plans?

Number 1 – hunger. You just never feel satisfied. The Gi Point Diet provides **all the food you need** to satisfy your hunger. We even order you to **eat snacks between meals**!

Number 2 – boring foods. You have to eat the very things you don't like. The Gi Point Diet lets **you eat normal foods**. You choose the foods you like. Just keep to the generous portions and daily points allowance and you'll lose weight. And if you go mad occasionally – hey, that's allowed for too!

Number 3 – keeping to it. Who wants to feel they're on a permanent diet?

The Gi Point Diet helps you stay on track with its tried and tested motivational tools. You're not 'on a diet' – you're changing your life, for the better, for good.

So, what's the secret? Get ready to be gripped! It includes strategies that *keep you focused* and *keep you full*. If you haven't had much success with other diets, then be prepared to succeed this time, with flying colours. Boost your self-belief: you can achieve the goals you seek – today, now.

Follow the quick tips and guidelines and see the results for yourself – in your clothes, in your new-found confidence and in the flattering comments of friends, family and partner. Eating the foods you like while watching the pounds slide away and your waist reappear has never been so easy.

And here's a great bonus. You don't have to read the whole book before you get going. Just turn to our Quick Start Guide on page 1 and you can begin the Gi Point Diet today, and take your first step towards becoming the person you want to be. Then, over the next few days, you can take your time to read through this book and discover how and why the Gi Point Diet really works. This is our little gift for you. The Gi Point Diet is your *big gift* to yourself!

This diet is about eating well. Chapter 9 is your

comprehensive guide to balanced nutrition. Here are the main benefits in a nutshell. The Gi Point Diet ...

- is simple, practical and flexible. It fits into your lifestyle – not the other way round.
- uses a blend of the latest scientific knowledge and traditional wisdom to ensure you eat healthily – and still lose weight.
- shows you how to avoid hunger pangs by eating the 'right carbs'.
- teaches you how to deal with emotional eating and other dieting hurdles – effortlessly!
- helps you become – and stay – motivated, by using insights that tap into the incredible power of your mind.

The result? You reach your target weight and size. And stay there!

NOTE: Glycaemic Index is an international ranking of foods, comparing the speed at which a particular food raises blood glucose levels. The Gi Point (GiP) system is designed specifically for this diet. It takes into account the glycaemic index and calorie density of foods, and encourages good nutrition. In this book, GiPs and 'points' mean the same thing.

PART ONE

A HEALTHY EATING PLAN

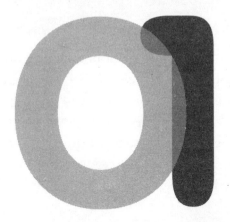

QUICK START GUIDE

So you want to get started straight away? Then you've come to the right place as this Quick Start Guide is designed for that purpose. However, it is essential that you read the rest of the book very soon to ensure you are following the plan correctly.

'A good beginning makes a good ending,' so the old proverb says. So we believe that a *great* beginning is bound to make a *great* ending. Give this short section your complete attention for the next few minutes – in particular the section entitled 'Five crucial minutes towards your goal' (page 4) – even if you're just browsing through this book. Otherwise come back later when you have a little more time. Ready?

The low-down on carbs

When you eat 'carbs' – or carbohydrate foods (such as bread, potatoes, pasta, cereals and sugary foods), the body digests it and converts it to glucose (a simple sugar). This raises the glucose level in your blood. Different carbs cause the blood glucose level to rise at different rates. Some cause a sharp rise in your blood glucose while others cause a gradual rise.

The Glycaemic Index (GI)

The Glycaemic Index (GI) is a way of ranking foods based on the rate at which they raise blood-glucose levels. Each food is given a number:

- Foods that raise blood glucose quickly have a high glycaemic index number. They are best kept to a minimum.
- Foods that raise blood glucose more slowly have a low glycaemic index number. These can help you lose weight because they make you feel full for longer.

Keeping your blood glucose levels more stable can improve your sensitivity to an important hormone in the body, called insulin. People who are overweight may be less sensitive to insulin, which makes you more prone to diabetes and possibly heart problems.

High-GI foods aren't necessarily bad foods. Neither are low-GI foods necessarily good foods. It is well recognised that GI alone is not sufficient. Hence the Gi Point Diet (aka The 'GiP' Diet).

The Gi Point Diet

The key to successful weight loss is to get the right mix of foods that ensure stable blood-glucose levels and take into account the calorie value of foods, while still providing the nutrients needed for optimal health. This is the unique feature of the Gi Point Diet. It does all the fancy calculating for you. This programme is an innovative way to choose the right carbs and stay in shape. It also boasts some of the best-kept motivation secrets and will-power boosters, as you'll see throughout the book.

What's the difference between the Gi Point Diet and a low-carb diet? Lots. But, in a nutshell, GiP is about choosing the right carbs; those carbs that are known to be healthy, like wholegrains, pulses, pasta, fruit and vegetables. In contrast, you get little of these on a low-carbohydrate diet. GiP encourages a wide variety of foods so that you are not missing out on key nutrients. Low-carb diets appear to restrict certain food groups. GiP encourages slow, steady and sustainable weight loss rather than rapid weight loss.

Many common food items have been given a certain number of Gi points (GiPs). These are listed in special tables in the book. Each day you have a certain number of points that you can use on the foods you want. You choose the foods, so you are in control of what you eat. You just need to follow certain guidelines and keep close to your allocated points each day. In no time, you'll learn how to make your points go further by choosing wisely, so you lose weight without going hungry. And that's basically it. All you do then is tweak here and there, as you get towards the new slimmer, trimmer and fitter you!

Five crucial minutes towards your goal

Think of a time when you really enjoyed yourself ... a holiday perhaps, a party, a sporting match or just a good night out. Okay? Now, in your mind, go back in time to that occasion ... And as you step into that place, take a moment or so to be there again ... Listen to the sounds – what do you hear? What pictures are you seeing? What are you feeling? Enjoy these feelings for a few seconds ...

Your mind makes sense of your reality through pictures, sounds and feelings, as we have just seen. Tastes and smells are important too. How does this help you to achieve your goal – for example a slim, trim, new you? Once your goal is clear, your attention automatically focuses on what you need. Your mind selects what it considers to be important in order to achieve the goal. This may include healthier food choices and physical activity as part of your everyday routine. Your energy flows where your attention goes. So what you think about, you bring into your life.

Let's now use this for your specific goal.

What is your goal or outcome?

Take a moment and answer this question as clearly as you can. And here's a big tip – state it in positive words, as something you want rather than something you don't want. Perhaps you really want to get into that bikini, or into your wedding dress. Maybe you want a flatter belly, perhaps a six-pack, or to drop a size, or simply to become trimmer and fitter. Whatever it is, take this time now and answer the question – what is your goal?

Now picture yourself as the person you want to become – the new you. How would you look? Imagine how you would be ... Perhaps healthy, fit, energetic, confident? What would you sound like? Be specific. What would you be saying? And how are you saying it? What are others saying about you? Hear their compliments. Connect with your new self now, give yourself a taster of what's to come ... And how are you feeling? Really step inside the new you and experience the feeling. Stay there for a few moments and enjoy it ...

A mentor once said:

'I don't start a task until I have decided what the end result is.'

We know from highly successful people that the goal then becomes just a formality. Now you too have decided what your end result is.

You are a human being, but it's easy to become influenced by others and get busy with too much stuff which turns you into a human doing! Before you know it, you can lose the plot and fit into somebody else's lifestyle. Now's the time to make different, inspiring choices, to live the life you **really** want, which is lurking within.

How are you feeling now? With your new, inspiring goal fresh in your mind? Please write it down as recommended in Step 1 below.

Congratulations, you are now formally on the programme.

The GiP Diet plan in 15 steps

Follow these steps and tick them off as you get them done.

Step 1: *Write down your goal and the date for reaching that goal.* The best way to keep to a healthy happy weight in the long term is to lose around 1 kg (2 lb) each week, so be realistic and your target weight is yours forever.

Also decide how you will know when you've achieved your goal. It may be something you'll see or hear yourself, or others, say. Or it could be how you'll feel. Put your goal up somewhere prominent so you can look at it often.

Step 2: *Weigh yourself either now or in the next couple of days.* Check out the BMI chart (page 49) to find a healthy weight for you. There are a couple of other vital measurements that would help you, such as waist measurements. If you want to know about this, turn to page 50. But now let's start to shed some pounds!

Step 3: *Enter the Start-it Phase* (first two weeks). The Gi Point Diet is split into three phases. Each has been carefully designed to guide you to your desired goal in an optimum way. It is important that you follow the instructions to reach your target weight and stay there. You are now starting the first phase of the Gi Point Diet – the Start-it Phase. This is designed to kick-start your weight loss, and is only suitable for the first two weeks. You are likely to lose weight reasonably quickly in this phase, but this initial weight loss is mostly water.

Step 4: *How many points for me?* Use the table below and read off the number of points you can have per day in the Start-it Phase. You are allowed to have food worth this many points each day (see page 36).

GiPs per day

	Start-it Phase (initial 2 weeks)	Lose-it Phase (until target)	Keep-it Phase (staying on target)
Women	17	20	23 or more
Men	22	25	28 or more

Plus, in addition to your daily GiPs, you can have 200 ml (⅓ pint) semi-skimmed milk each day. What's more, if you fancy a tipple, women can include 7 units of alcohol each week, and men 10 units per week (see page 192).

Step 5: *Follow the guidelines.* The Gi Point Diet includes some basic guidelines. These are called the 'GiP Rules'. They are designed to help you lose weight, keep feeling full and get a wide variety of nutrients needed for overall good health. Some are non-dietary – this isn't just a diet, it's a fun way to be. The complete GiP rules are listed at the end of this chapter. Copy them out and display them in a prominent place. Put them on, say, the fridge door or on your desk at work, so you can look at them often until they become second nature.

Step 6: *Eat three meals and three snacks every day* (**GiP Rule 1**). Try to have your main meal at lunchtime and a lighter meal in the evening. Here are a couple of examples of an ideal day during the Lose-it Phase for:

Women		Men	
(20-points-a-day plan)		(25-points-a-day plan)	
Breakfast	4 GiPs	Breakfast	5 GiPs
Mid-morning	1½ GiPs	Mid-morning	2 GiPs
Lunch	6 GiPs	Lunch	8 GiPs
Mid-afternoon	1½ GiPs	Mid-afternoon	2 GiPs
Dinner	5 GiPs	Dinner	6 GiPs
Evening snack	2 GiPs	Evening snack	2 GiPs

Step 7: *Stock up on basic low-GiP foods.* Use our Smart Shopping lists (see page 57) to help you choose. Having these foods handy will make it much easier to enjoy the diet early on. So just photocopy some of the shopping pages and call in at the supermarket on your way home.

Step 8: *Start simple – use the ready-made meal/menu plans provided* (pages 82–97). You might also like to sample the recipes (see page 129). Their points values are given alongside so you don't have to work them out. There are meal plans for:

● Breakfasts
● Light and main meals
● Snacks

Or make up your own meals from the Gi Point Table (see page 284). Or mix and match between the menu plans and the table. It's all about flexibility.

Step 9: *Keep as close as you can to your daily GiPs* (**GiP Rule 2**). Don't use up all your points by lunchtime! Balance your points – you'll soon be an ace at budgeting with your daily GiPs so you're not in the red before sunset. If at times you think you may have a high-GiP meal, then mix a low-GiP carb with it, such as salad, to bring down the overall Glycaemic Index of your meal (see page 40). GI research doesn't include all foods so sometimes there is no GiP value. Keep such choices to a minimum.

Step 10: *Have one 'meal carb' at each meal, and 2–3 servings of protein each day* (**GiP Rule 3**). Meal carbs are carbohydrate foods that have some starch. They are clearly marked in the Gi Point Table. You need them because this diet is not a 'low-carb' diet, it's a 'right-carb' diet. Choose 2–3 servings of protein foods (such as lean meat, fish, eggs, beans), keeping to the amounts suggested in the Gi Point Table. This will help you at a glance to balance your meals and to keep to GiP Rule 5 at the same time.

Step 11: *Picture your plate in quarters and fill two quarters with vegetables (v, v), one quarter with protein (p) and one quarter with carbs (c).* Here's how you'll remember this: veggie, veggie, protein, carbs (**GiP Rule 4**).

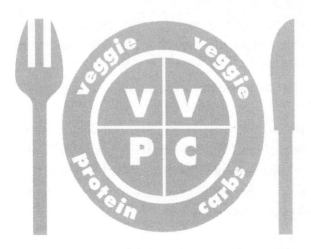

Step 12: *Have at least one low-GiP food at each meal and always have a snack* (**GiP Rule 5**). Making sure you have a snack helps to make the Gi Point Diet work. It keeps that blood-glucose level steady and curbs hunger pangs.

Step 13: *Imagine the new you every day – a past photograph will help* (**GiP Rule 6**). It's not all about what's on your plate. The key is to examine what's going on in your mind.

- *Picture* yourself as the person that you most want to be – the 'new' you. See the picture in as much detail as you can, as if it has already happened. See yourself with people who are supportive and fun. Like laughter, it's infectious! See yourself being able to fit into your favourite jeans.

- *Hear* the comments others are making to you, now that you've achieved your goal. Hear their congratulations.
- *Feel* the positivity of your success and how these feelings and emotions make you feel so great about yourself. Feel that enhanced sense of energy and inner confidence growing. Put up a photograph of how you want to look – the new you – somewhere you'll see it often. That will spur you on even more.

Step 14: *Have at least two 10-minute bursts of moderate-intensity physical activity every day* (**GiP Rule 7**). Being GiP-fit means doing only two daily 10-minute bursts of exercise. For example, walk more and briskly, use the stairs more, get off one stop early and walk, exercise at home. The possibilities are endless. You could, of course, go swimming, go to the gym, do aerobics, or take up a hobby like badminton. Aim to feel slightly breathless and warm during your 10 minutes. (You should not be so breathless that you cannot hold a conversation.)

So decide now what you will do and when. Better to start something small today than wait for something bigger tomorrow. You can always change later. Get someone else to join you if you can.

Step 15: *Choose a balanced day by having a variety of foods from the different food groups* (**GiP Rule 8**). You can find

> If you are not used to exercise, do check with your doctor before you start.

out more about the food groups in Chapter 9, Eating for Complete Health.

NOTE: These are the basic 15 steps. What next? There are two more things you need to know.

Enter the Lose-it Phase (from week three)

You move on to this phase after the first two weeks. Here you can eat more. Check out the 'Points per day' table above and read off the number of points (GiPs) you have per day in the Lose-it column for your sex. You should now have more points in a day than before and therefore be able to eat more.

Remind yourself of the 15 steps. Start with the suggested number of GiPs and check your progress at the end of week three. You should be losing ½–1 kg (1–2 lb) per week. Don't be tempted to lose more – research shows that if you try to lose weight too quickly, you are more likely to put the weight back on, as with so many diets. So keep it slow and steady. Also losing weight too quickly can be harmful in the long term.

Check and correct your daily GiPs if appropriate

If you lose more than ½–1 kg (2 lb) per week, increase your daily GiPs by 3 points or so (you will then eat more and slow down your weight loss).

If you don't lose ½–1 kg (1–2 lb) per week, decrease your daily GiPs by 3 points or so (you will then eat less and lose more weight).

Having more GiPs during Lose-it simply means you can eat more. Not only does this feel fab, it helps you to avoid hunger too. Feeling full and including more daily GiPs means that this phase fits more easily into your lifestyle.

Enter the Keep-it Phase

You have reached your target weight. Well done! Reward yourself and enjoy the new you. At this point you enter the Keep-it Phase. Once you've reached a more desirable weight, the GiP system helps you keep hold of your new lifestyle. You are in charge of how many GiPs you need to keep you slim and fit.

Look at the 'GiPs per day' table on page 8 and find out the number of GiPs you have per day in the Keep-it column for your sex. And use that as your new daily points total. Again, check your weight regularly to make sure it's stable. If it's not, adjust your daily GiPs a little, as described in the Lose-it Phase. Enjoy!

The key to long-term weight loss: lose ½–1 kg (1–2 lb) per week and no more!

Caution

- This chapter gives you just some information to get you started. It is not designed to give you everything you need. We strongly advise you to read and understand the whole book.

- If you are not sure about your general well-being, see your doctor before you start this or any other diet or any exercise programme.

The GiP Rules

GiP Rule 1: Eat three meals and three snacks every day (page 37).

GiP Rule 2: Keep as close as you can to your daily GiPs (page 40).

GiP Rule 3: Have one 'meal carb' at each meal, and 2–3 servings of protein each day (page 42).

GiP Rule 4: Picture your plate in quarters and fill two quarters with vegetables (v, v), one quarter with protein (p) and one quarter with carbs (c). Here's how you'll remember this: veggie, veggie, protein, carbs (page 42).

GiP Rule 5: Have at least one low-GiP food at each meal and always have a snack (page 24).

GiP Rule 6: Imagine the new you every day – a past photograph will help (page 237).

GiP Rule 7: Have at least two 10-minute bursts of moderate-intensity physical activity every day (page 203).

GiP Rule 8: Choose a balanced day by having a variety of foods from the different food groups (page 158).

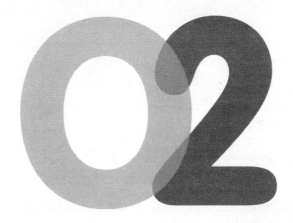

WHAT IS GI?

The fuss about carbohydrate

Flick through any newspaper to see all the conflicting info on carbohydrate foods: 'avoid wheat', 'starchy foods are fattening', or 'pasta is the best food ever invented'. How do you know what's best? Well, let's review some of the issues here.

When you eat a carbohydrate food (such as bread, potatoes, pasta, cereals and sugary foods), the body digests it and converts it to glucose (a simple sugar); this can then be used for energy. As the carbohydrate gets converted to glucose, the glucose level in your blood rises.

We know different foods cause the blood glucose to rise at different rates. Some foods cause a sharp rise in your blood-glucose levels, and these are best kept to a minimum. Other foods cause a gradual rise in blood glucose levels, and these can help you lose weight. So the speed at which carbohydrate foods are digested plays an important part in losing weight and in over-all health, as we will now see.

The Glycaemic Index

The Glycaemic Index (GI) ranks foods according to the speed at which they raise blood-glucose levels. Each food is given a number:

- Foods that raise blood glucose quickly are said to have a high Glycaemic Index.
- Foods that raise blood glucose more slowly have a low Glycaemic Index.

Here's a simplified way of looking at this:

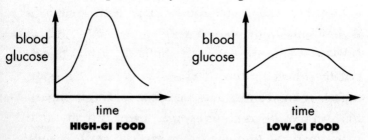

The Glycaemic Index has been studied around the world for years and the findings have been published extensively in medical journals (for Research, References and Further Reading see page 338).

Filling not fattening

So how does GI help us? Well, there are two huge benefits. The first good news is for slimmers because the more stable your blood-glucose levels, the less hungry you will feel.

Foods that cause sharp rises in blood glucose are best kept to a minimum, because they don't fill you up as much, leaving you more likely to reach for the biscuit barrel. Foods that cause a rapid rise in blood glucose have a high GI, so the key is to regularly choose more foods with low GIs (we'll see how later).

The main thing to remember is that low-GI foods are digested slowly and cause a slow and steady rise in blood glucose, followed by a steady fall. Slower digestion helps to make you feel full for longer, and so delays hunger pangs. In this book we call these foods the 'right carbs'.

And here's a bonus – the effect of a low-GI meal can run on to the following meal, which helps keep blood glucose more even throughout the day. This, in turn, helps you control hunger pangs.

This principle, though complex, is based on how you digest food and how a particular food acts within your body to help you feel full for longer.

In 2000, DS Ludwig conducted a review of the effects of GI on obesity and concluded that 'To date at least 16 studies have examined the effects of GI on appetite and all but one have demonstrated an increase in satiety, delayed hunger return and

Tip: Keep starchy foods as whole as possible and avoid mashing or processing as this can raise the GI.

reduced food intake following low GI foods than following high GI foods' (see Research, References and Further Reading, page 338).

The second benefit is that choosing foods that raise your blood glucose slowly helps to prevent or minimise diabetes and obesity. Research has also shown that people who have an overall low-GI diet have a lower incidence of heart disease, and lower-GI diets have been associated with improved levels of 'good' cholesterol too.

A lot of this is common sense: 'whole' foods, such as wholegrains, and foods high in a particular type of fibre called 'soluble fibre', such as kidney beans, take longer to be broken down by the body compared to, say, a sugary drink. Therefore grains and beans cause a slower rise in blood glucose. These foods have a relatively low GI. Filling up on low-GI carbohydrate foods in meals and snacks means there's less room for fat, so when you're watching your weight, you're also helping to keep your calorie intake down. The trick is to choose right carbs rather than avoiding carbs altogether.

So, is it simply a matter of knowing your GIs?

The GI only tells you how quickly or slowly a food raises blood glucose. But foods with a high GI are not bad foods. Compare potato crisps, which have a medium GI, to a baked potato, which has a high GI. Interestingly, white pitta bread has a lower GI than wholemeal bread – could you ever have guessed that? And some biscuits and cakes have a lower GI than bread – does this mean we should fill up on these?

The key to using GI successfully in weight loss is to get the right mix of foods. This will not only ensure more stable blood-glucose levels, it will also take into account the calorie value of the foods and help you obtain the wide variety of nutrients needed for overall good health. This is the unique feature of the GiP system. It is a revolutionary way to choose the right carbs and stay in shape forever. This diet programme has another plus – it is supported by some of the best-kept motivation secrets and will-power boosters.

It is cumbersome, impractical and not sensible to use the GI in isolation. The Gi Point Diet does all the fancy calculating for you, taking note of the calories and GI, giving you a simple method that you can use with confidence.

Let's take another example. Chocolate has a medium GI – so does this mean you can have your cake and eat it? As always, there is a place for chocolate, though it's advisable to limit it to small amounts at the end of a high-fibre meal. The fibre helps to slow down the digestion. Chocolate may have a low GI, but since it's also a high-fat, high-calorie food, this isn't the way the Glycaemic Index was intended to be used. Choosing foods with a low GI – as well as those that are low in saturated fat – makes good sense. And since we eat meals, not single foods, eating mainly low-GI foods along with a few high-GI foods will ensure you're being practical and realistic and yet keeping to an overall medium GI in your diet.

Are carbs cool – or not?

It was once believed that all starchy carbohydrate foods, such as bread, rice and potatoes, were digested slowly, causing a gradual increase in blood-sugar levels. However, it is now known that many starchy foods, such as certain types of rice and breads, are digested very rapidly and absorbed quickly. They are high-GI carbs.

In short, some carbs are cool and others may be best swapped for alternatives, even if it's the same basic food, just cooked or prepared differently.

There are some foods, such as beans and lentils, that would seem to have an obviously lower GI. But the way that they are cooked or processed can also affect the GI. So, for example, dried kidney beans boiled have a very low GI, but scoop them out of a can and you'll find that the GI reaches a medium classification. An orange has a low GI, but squeezing it into orange juice raises the GI. In contrast, the acids in lime or lemon juice can help to lower the overall GI of a meal. A serving of peeled boiled potato has a medium GI, but make this into mash and the GI reaches the 'high' category (even higher for instant mash). So, the more mashed up or processed a food is, the higher its GI is likely to be. Use the Point Table (page 284) to give you a more accurate assessment of how a food will affect your blood-glucose levels – and your weight – rather than just guessing.

What, no more high GIs? Ever?

If you only ate low-GI foods, you might lose weight, but you wouldn't stick to it for long. And, as with many other diets, the weight would creep back on again. The key is to enjoy what you eat, choosing foods that fit in with who you are, your lifestyle, your likes and dislikes, and so on. Although foods with a high GI do not offer favourable effects on blood glucose, we're only human. So why deny yourself the odd high-GI food? Indeed these foods may be good for you in other ways. Take bread, for example: multi-grain bread has a lower GI than other breads, but what if you detest the stuff? Do you go without bread and crave for it every time you pass the bakery? Not on the GiP plan, you don't. You make choices based on what else you're eating. You might opt for white bread, a higher-GI food, but then whack some baked beans (a medium-GI food) on top to lower the overall blood-glucose response – sorted!

Meal combos

When you mix foods together in a meal, this affects the GI – and it isn't simply a case of taking the average GI of the individual foods to find out the overall GI of the meal. However, you can predict the GI of a meal using a special formula. The Gi Point table has already used this formula to calculate a selection of breakfasts, light meals and recipes for main meals, so you can have a more accurate point value for these mixed meals. It would be impossible to calculate all possible meal and food combinations, so use the sample mixed meals as often as you like and mix and match your other food choices with this. The key to remember is to choose low-GiP carbs at each meal or snack. Then you know you're doing the best you can whilst having variety and freedom of choice.

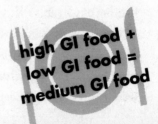

high GI food + low GI food = medium GI food

Can we play the guessing game?

Popcorn has a much higher GI than sweetcorn. Popcorn is high in fibre and protein and is a great snack food, but because the GI is considered to be high, you'll notice that it's been given more points than some other snack foods (see page 302). However, if you do opt for crunching the corn, you could try making your own so that it's not cooked in a lot of oil and smothered in salt. Eating popcorn with a low-GI food, such as nuts, also helps, so long as you're not downing it by the bowlful! (See the recipe for Chilli Peanut Popcorn, page 137).

Is GI on a food label?

Not yet. On its own the GI is not that helpful, as we have explained above. Some low-GI foods can be high in fat, so the Glycaemic Index value on a label may be counter-productive. However, the good news is that the GiP system, which takes other factors into account, could be something that manufacturers adopt, since it allows consumers to make more of an informed choice. There are GI values for foods such as Kellogg's cereals, Ryvita and Nesquik. But since the GI value alone is not very helpful, it would not be appropriate for manufacturers of these foods to use the GI on a label without providing more information. Supermarkets such as Sainsbury's have taken the GI message on board by producing a leaflet on the subject. Tesco are looking into putting the GI on their label. So who knows where the GiPs will end up?

Do all foods have a GI?

No. And since low-GI foods are good choices, you might assume that those with no GI would be better for you – not true. Many non-carbohydrate foods won't raise blood glucose, so they won't have a GI figure. But they might not be good for weight loss. Take fried steak or lard, for example. The Gi Point Diet takes weight loss and good nutrition into account so that you are generally choosing GI-free foods that are lower in fat, especially saturated fat. In this way, you are more likely to choose low GI foods in the right context.

And the calculation of GI requires careful laboratory analysis – not all foods have been analysed, even if they do contain carbs. Some branded foods, such as Kellogg's All Bran, have been analysed, but to avoid promoting specific brands, generic names are used in some cases.

Other benefits of the Gi way of eating

● Foods that have a low GI are often high in fibre. Choosing those that are low in fat, too, such as

Low-GI foods can help you control your appetite by making you feel fuller for longer, with the result that you eat less.

pasta, will fill you up and cut down on calories, helping you to maintain a healthy weight.

- People who are overweight and/or have diabetes are more prone to coronary heart disease. A diet based on low- or medium-GI foods, as part of a healthy lifestyle, can be particularly useful in helping to reduce the risk of heart disease in these people. Some low-GI foods, such as those high in soluble fibre (beans, peas and lentils) can also help reduce blood cholesterol.

- People who have a condition called reactive hypoglycaemia can incorporate a range of low-GI foods to help stabilise their blood-glucose levels.

- The right combination of low- and high-GI foods can help sports performance. Low-GI foods, such as pasta, are great for 'carbohydrate loading' (energy storage) before a sports event, and high-GI foods, such as a glucose drink, provide fast-release carbohydrate, quickly replacing glucose in the bloodstream after an event.

- GiP is a godsend for the condition Syndrome X – see page 29.

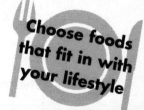

Choose foods that fit in with your lifestyle

A rough guideline – foods high in soluble fibre will have a lower GI; keeping starchy foods whole can reduce their GI; eating veg keeps the GI low.

Ten GiP tips

1 Have one low-GI food at each meal or snack.

2 Choose breakfast cereals based on wholegrains, such as oats (porridge for example).

3 Opt for grainy breads made with whole seeds, barley and oats, instead of white or brown bread.

4 Wheat-based pasta, sweet potato and basmati rice are cool – enjoy them regularly and check portion sizes on the Gi Point Table (page 284).

5 Dairy foods are low GI and high in calcium – have reduced-fat milk and low-fat yoghurt two or three times a day.

6 Eat more beans, lentils and peas. Toss them into stews and casseroles, or simply spice them up with lemon juice and chilli for a snack.

7 Go for whole fruits rather than fruit juices. The lower-GI ones include apples, dried apricots, cherries, grapefruit, grapes, oranges, peaches, pears, plums and firm bananas.

8 Under is better than over: choose foods that are under-processed, whole or just cooked, rather than overcooked (such as mushy veg and mash).

9 Go for the fibre fill-up (see page 162). It helps slow the digestion and absorption of starchy foods.

10 Most vegetables and fruits have a low-GI rating, and are low in calories and fat – they are your best friends.

Syndrome X

You might have come across the strange term 'Syndrome X' and wondered what on earth it was. It sounds like something rather sinister from a science fiction movie but it actually refers to a collection of medical conditions that can occur together in the same person. These include:

- Central obesity, or an 'apple shape', which means a waist measurement of more than 94 cm (37 in) for men and more than 80 cm (32 in) for women.
- Poor blood-glucose control.
- High blood pressure.
- Abnormal blood-fat levels including raised triglycerides (a type of fat in the blood) and low HDL (the good form of cholesterol).
- 'Sticky blood' with an increased tendency to form dangerous clots.

If you have three or more of these conditions, you may very well have Syndrome X and should seek proper medical diagnosis. Each of the above characteristics

There is evidence that a low-GI diet can help control diabetes, aid weight loss, lower blood fats, and improve the body's sensitivity to insulin, by keeping blood-glucose levels more stable.

makes you more prone to heart disease and having more than one of them increases your risk considerably. However, by consciously choosing to make changes to your lifestyle today, you could reduce the risk of developing these conditions.

What's insulin resistance got to do with it?

Syndrome X is sometimes referred to as 'metabolic syndrome' or 'insulin resistance syndrome'. It seems to run in families. Current thinking is that all the conditions associated with the disorder arise from one main cause – insulin resistance (IR).

If you are less sensitive to insulin – the hormone responsible for allowing glucose to leave the bloodstream and enter your cells – you can become insulin resistant. As a result, an organ in your body called the pancreas reacts by trying to produce more insulin, leading to high circulating levels of the hormone in the blood. If insulin resistance becomes severe, a condition called type 2 diabetes can develop.

How common is it?

Syndrome X seems to be very common in the Western

world. Estimates from the USA and Scandinavia suggest that 10–25 per cent of adults show some degree of insulin resistance. So, in a room of 100 people, at least 10 are likely to be affected. Scary! Syndrome X is sometimes said to be 'silent' since most people who have it are unaware of it.

People at risk of developing Syndrome X include those with:

- obesity;
- a family history of type 2 diabetes;
- a history of diabetes during pregnancy (gestational diabetes).

What can you do if you have Syndrome X?

Research has shown that both insulin resistance and the symptoms of Syndrome X can be improved by lifestyle changes, including physical activity levels and diet. There is some research suggesting a diet based mainly on foods with a low Glycaemic Index may improve insulin sensitivity. The good news is that these lifestyle approaches, if successfully adopted, are very effective in reducing the risk of developing heart disease and type 2 diabetes. The GiP programme dovetails with these lifestyle changes.

Lifestyle guidelines for Syndrome X

- Take regular physical activity – something such as brisk walking.

- Cut down on the amount of fat (and especially saturated fat) that you eat.
- Replace saturated fats with mono- and polyunsaturated fats from vegetable sources and fish.
- Eat low-GI and fibre-rich foods, fruit and vegetables.
- Keep body weight to within 20 per cent of ideal targets.
- Drink alcohol only in moderation.
- Give up smoking.

The most important product of your life is you

Learn to nurture and nourish yourself by making healthy choices in the foods you eat and the amount of regular physical activity you take. This is vital in building a caring relationship with yourself. If you don't like yourself, you're less likely to care for yourself, let alone others. Caring for your body will encourage you to put the right foods into it.

Are you a Real Gipper?

Question:

How do you choose your foods?

Choice 1: I seek out and choose foods with low GiPs as often as I can.

Consequently, you are making excellent choices for

more steady blood glucose, one of the most important aims of a Real Gipper.

Choice 2: I make food choices irrespective of whether they're high or low GiPs.

Consequently, you are less aware of the effects that different foods have on your blood glucose, making it more difficult to keep within your daily Gi Point Diet.

Choice 3: I choose more foods that are high in GiPs because I like them more.

Consequently, your blood-glucose levels are more likely to be unstable, so hunger pangs are more likely to occur.

Results:

Choice 1: Congratulations! Making these kinds of conscious choices will enrich your life by giving you a sense of achievement. This, in turn, is likely to keep you motivated and up-beat in your mental approach and attitude.

Choice 2: Ignorance is mental poverty! This could have direct consequences, preventing you from achieving your goal. Enjoy finding out about the choices that exist and take responsibility for your life and its results. After all, you're in control.

Choice 3: You can start by making different choices

today, knowing that this will get you nearer to your ultimate 'new you' goal. Short term, many will opt for instant gratification, but this can be at the risk of creating long-term issues for themselves. Make up your mind to make the change here and now – and then stick with it.

So be a Real Gipper – and choose in line with the new you.

Summary

- Fill up on low-GI carbs at meals, thereby making less room for fat and helping to keep the calories down.
- Choose 'whole foods' that take longer to be broken down by the body.
- The GiP Diet facilitates more stable glucose levels, and a calorie-controlled eating plan, integrated into a healthy eating and activity programme.

03

THE DIET PROGRAMME

What's so sexy about GiP?

Dieting using the Glycaemic Index alone doesn't necessarily mean you'll lose weight, because you could be filling up on low-GI but high-calorie foods. The Gi Point Diet importantly takes calories into account so that achieving your target weight is all part of the plan. Top this with tried and tested behavioural and will-power tips and you end up with an ingenious cocktail of weight-loss strategies.

The beauty of the GiP system is that the experts have done all the calculating for you, so all you have to do is add up the points you're eating for the day. The system automatically takes into account:

- the Glycaemic Index value of the listed foods
- calories
- portion sizes that will fill you up as well as help you lose weight steadily
- healthy eating strategies

This makes the diet healthy, slimming and practical. How easy is that?

GiPs uniquely incorporate the Glycaemic Index, calories as well as good nutritional guidelines which you cannot achieve using the GI alone.

The GiP system

The system is really very easy. Food items have been given a certain number of GI points (GiPs). Now, imagine that you're given a pot of points each day, which you can spend on the foods you want to eat. Just as you would spend money to buy food from a store, here you can choose which foods you spend your points on that day. So you are in control of what you eat.

Keep as close as you can to your daily allowance of GiPs, and each new day you get another set of points to spend. It's just like going to the cash machine, but here, the points come to you.

You'll learn how to make your points go further by choosing wisely, so you lose weight without going hungry. What's more, you even get a bonus – you follow some basic tips and you'll even end up having a nutritious and balanced diet without thinking too much about it. So you'll not only lose weight, but you'll also be looking after that all-important tool in your life – your body.

All this will help you learn new skills and behaviours. They will soon become automatic – actions that you do almost without thinking, like driving a car or swimming. This soon becomes a lifestyle change that lasts forever!

So, are you ready for the new slimmer, trimmer and fitter you? ... Then let's get started.

GI is based on how foods affect your blood glucose levels (Chapter 2) so one of the keys to GiP eating is to eat regular meals and snacks. In fact, you're eating six times a day! Simply spread out your points to suit your lifestyle and tastes, making sure you distribute your GiPs evenly throughout the day. Aim to have your main meal at lunchtime and a lighter meal in the evening.

For example, if you are on the 20-points-a-day plan (for women), your ideal day might look like this:

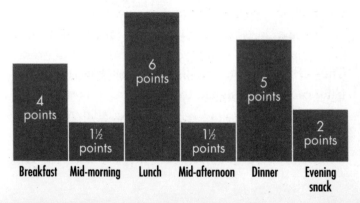

And a 25-points-a-day plan (for men) might look like this:

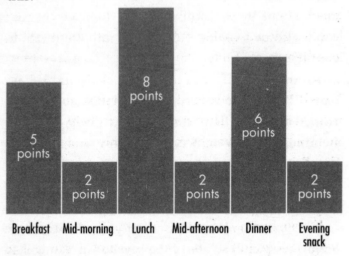

GiP Rule 1:
Eat three meals and three snacks every day.

The GiP phases

Start-it ⇨ Lose-it ⇨ Keep-it

The GiP diet is split into three phases. Each phase has been carefully designed to guide you to your desired goal in an optimal way. It is important that you follow the instructions below to reach your target weight and stay there.

Start-it Phase: The first phase, Start-it, is designed to kick-start your weight loss, but is only appropriate for the first two weeks. During this phase you are likely to lose weight reasonably quickly. As with any weight-loss plan, most of the initial weight loss is just water.

Lose-it Phase: The second phase, Lose-it, allows you more daily GiPs. This is designed to help you (eat more and) lose weight more steadily and sensibly. The British Dietetic Association recommends that the ideal rate of weight loss is around 0.5–1 kg (1–2 lb) per week.

If you opt for fewer GiPs, you'll probably lose weight more quickly. But research shows that trying to lose weight too quickly is not effective in keeping the weight off permanently. You are more likely to put the weight back on, as happens with many other diets. So keep it slow and steady, especially since losing weight too quickly can be harmful in the long term.

Having more GiPs during the Lose-it phase simply means you can eat more. Not only does this feel fab, it helps you to avoid hunger too. Feeling full and including more daily GiPs means that this phase fits more easily into your lifestyle.

The key to long-term weight loss: lose 0.5–1 kg (1–2 lb) per week and no more!

Keep-it Phase: Once you've reached a more desirable weight, the GiP system helps you keep hold of your new lifestyle. You are in charge of how many GiPs you need to keep you slim and fit.

How many GiPs for me?

In general, women are likely to lose an appropriate and steady amount of weight on 20 points per day, and 25 points a day is likely to suit men best. Use the table below to work out your daily GiPs. The calories you need to keep to in order to lose weight slowly and successfully depend on your age, weight and activity levels. However, this is a useful starting point for new Gippers:

	Start-it Phase (initial 2 weeks) GiPs per day	Lose-it Phase (until target) GiPs per day	Keep-it Phase (staying on target) GiPs per day
Women	17	20	23 or more
Men	22	25	28 or more

Be wise with your GiPs

If you gobble a couple of croissants for breakfast (12 points), a slice of cake mid-morning (6 points), and a sausage and mustard sandwich at lunch (around 9 points), then you know you have already blown it –

GiP Rule 2:
Keep as close as you can to your daily GiPs.

with nothing left for dinner! The key is to get smart by balancing your points. You'll soon be an ace at budgeting with your daily GiPs so that you're not in the red before sunset. Get into the habit of checking that you have enough GiPs left for dinner and the rest of the day.

Many meals and snacks (for example, those taken at breakfast, mid-morning and lunch) are habitual. Our choice of foods for these three eating sessions are often very similar. So, it's likely that you will soon get to know how many points you have left for the evening. You might choose to have a different distribution of points at the weekends, which is okay.

Since the aim is to keep your blood-glucose levels more or less steady throughout the day, having a rough guide to the number of points per meal or snack can be very helpful.

There will be times when only a high-GiP meal will do – and that's fine. Simply mix in a low-GiP carb (see page 24). This helps you to lower the overall glycaemic effect of the meal (for more on this, see Chapter 2). And if on occasion you don't know the GiP value of a meal, watch your portion size and add a low-GiP carb to it, just as a safeguard.

If at times you think you may have a high-GiP meal, then mix it with a low-GiP carb such as salad, to bring down the overall Glycaemic Index of your meal.

Picture your plate

Remember GiP Rule 4: Picture your plate in quarters. Two parts are to be filled with the veggies and/or salad, one for the meat, fish, pulses, etc., and the last quarter is for the starchy food or 'meal carb' like potatoes, pasta or rice.

In this way, you will instinctively be keeping to healthier proportions. Try thinking of meals as two veg plus meat, rather than meat and two veg. The vegetables are best treated as an integral part of the meal. Having your plate piled up with veg and salad is a great way to make sure you get a range of vitamins and minerals. You'll also find that most of these foods are either GiP-free or very low in points, so they'll fill you up and keep you trim. When it comes

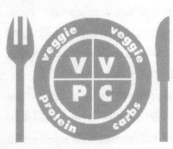

to carbohydrate, base meals and snacks on low-GiP carbs. Pasta and grainy breads fill you up and have a lower GI, so choose them often.

Choose a balanced day

Remember GiP Rule 8: Choose a balanced day by having a variety of foods from the different food groups.

Any dieting plan must encourage an overall balance of healthy foods. Details of the different food groups and nutrients are dealt with in Chapter 9 – Eating for Complete Health. For now, use the following guidelines as a checklist to make sure you get the balance right. Each day:

- Eat three meals and three snacks; keep fatty and sugary choices to a minimum.
- Have a 'meal carb' at each meal.
- Choose 2–3 portions of protein foods each day (such as lean meat, fish, eggs, cheese and beans), keeping to the amounts suggested in the Gi Point Table.
- Eat at least five portions of fruit and vegetables.
- Remember to picture your plate in quarters and to fill two quarters with vegetables (v, v), one quarter with protein (p) and one quarter with carbs (c) (veggie, veggie, protein, carbs).
- Drink 6–8 glasses of fluid (such as water, low-calorie drinks, herbal teas, milk, tea, coffee).
- Have a free daily allowance of 200 ml (⅓ pint) of semi-skimmed milk (an extra ½ point) in addition to milk with your breakfast cereal.
- Alcohol – no more than seven units for women and 10 units for men per week; this is in addition to your daily points (an optional bonus!). It's better to

> **GiP Rule 5:**
> Have at least one low-GiP carb at each meal and always have a snack.

drink less, though, and make sure you distribute your alcohol intake throughout the week.

Forcing yourself to have a snack may seem a bit pointless, but it is one of the foundations of the GiP system. Having a snack between meals helps to keep your blood-glucose level steady.

The foods and their points

GI only applies to carbohydrate foods. Not all foods have been analysed by the researchers, even if they do contain carbs. So it is not possible to know the GiPs of every food. However, the Gi Point Table includes a wide range of everyday foods so you can enjoy variety and flavour at home, at work and when eating out.

And since mixed meals have a different GI to individual foods, the meal combos in the table offer you a more accurate points value, based on predicted blood-glucose response.

Non-carbohydrate foods (such as meat and cheese) have been given a points value based on a Glycaemic Index of zero, as defined by international research (page 345). You'll note that fatty meats and some other high-saturated-fat foods have not been listed – it's best to keep these to a minimum.

Some branded foods, such as Kellogg's All Bran, have been analysed, but to avoid promoting any specific brands, the Gi Point Table does not give you the brand name.

GiP-free foods

There are certain foods that are so low in GiPs that you can enjoy them freely. Yes … they don't count towards your daily GiP allowance – you can have them for free!

You can eat some of these as much as you like, and others have a specified portion size. Check the Gi Point Table for a large selection of these delights.

Low-GiP carbs

Use these foods to make up your daily points wherever possible. By choosing low-GiP foods, you'll get more food for your points! Again, check out the Gi Point Table for details.

What about ready meals and eating out?

You'll notice that there are some ready meals in the Gi Point Table. As mentioned above, if the Glycaemic

You needn't avoid any food, simply think about how you can make it better. And if you can't, ask yourself whether there's another choice you could make.

Index of a meal has not been specified by researchers, then we don't know the points value. Try to keep to the foods for which we do know the points, but use your common sense too. It's far better to eat fresh foods, but there will be days when only food in a box will do and there isn't a points value – just don't go overboard. Maybe keep it to once a week, and mix in a low-GiP food, such as vegetables or a salad, to lower the overall glycaemic effect.

As for eating out, just turn to page 111 for a sack of GiP tips.

How to eat

Here are some clever ideas which encourage you to make small changes to the way you eat, which in turn can help keep you trim. Try one at a time and slowly build up till you can tick them all off.

- Treat everything you eat as a meal. Sit down, ideally at a dinner table rather than in front of the TV. Aim to sit upright.
- Have a break from whatever you're doing when you choose to have a snack.

- Avoid eating your lunch at your desk. And if you do have a snack at the PC, just relax your hands, move back a little and enjoy every mouthful.
- Have planned meals and snacks. If you simply nibble a bit here and there, note that this may influence your blood glucose, so it's better to keep to your three meals and three snacks a day.
- Put your cutlery down when you've taken in a mouthful. It allows space for chewing your food well, having a drink and engaging in conversation. Chewing slowly and eating at a steady pace can also reduce bloating and improve digestion.

What if the weight just falls off?

That's great! Or is it? Weigh yourself once a week – choose a day that suits you. Mondays may not be the best day if you're an indulgent weekender! You are likely to lose more than 1 kg (2 lb) during Start-it, especially if you keep to all the GiP rules. However, if at the end of week three you are still losing more than 1 kg (2 lb) a week, simply add a few more points (say, 3 points) until the weight loss becomes more slow and

As always, if you're concerned about your weight loss or anything else in your diet, consult your GP, who may refer you to a dietitian.

steady. You are the best judge of how many GiPs you need for an ideal rate of weight loss. It's best not to get tempted into keeping to a low-points diet just so that the weight rolls off – you are then less likely to keep the weight off in the long run.

What's my target weight?

So you're committed to keeping to the plan and to enjoying your new easy lifestyle that allows you to eat what you like so long as you keep to some basic guidelines. But how do you know what your ideal weight is? And is it more helpful to think of a 'happy weight' for you?

Body mass index

The body mass index (BMI) is one of the techniques used by doctors and dietitians to assess whether you are a healthy weight. To calculate your BMI, take your weight (in kilograms) and divide this by your height (in metres squared):

$$\text{BMI} = \frac{\text{Weight (kg)}}{\text{Height (m)}^2}$$

The most desirable range is a BMI of between 20 and 24. A larger BMI is an indication of being overweight.

The chart opposite will help you to work out just how much weight you need to lose to be within a

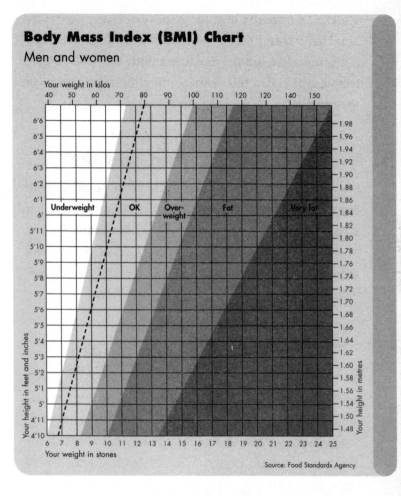

Body Mass Index (BMI) Chart

Men and women

Source: Food Standards Agency

healthy range. Plot your height (without shoes) on the left-hand axis. Plot your weight (without clothes) on the horizontal axis. Make a straight line from each mark and note where the two lines meet. This will show you what your BMI is – your target weight will be in the 'healthy weight range'. Aim for the higher end of this range for now. Once you have maintained your new weight for a few months, you can then aim for a lower weight by reducing your GiPs, so long as you keep within the healthy weight range – don't go overboard!

Take the carrier bag test

As you lose weight, whether it's half a pound or two pounds, put something of the same weight into a carrier or shopping bag. As you continue to lose weight, add other items (such as a packet of sugar for every 1 kg/2 lb) and just see and feel the weight pile up in the bag while it drops off your body.

The 'fruit salad' theory

Are you an 'apple-shape' or a 'pear-shape'?

This may sound unimportant, but in fact sound scientific theories have been formulated using this information. Putting weight on around the tummy ('central obesity') is said to be associated with resistance to insulin (see page 30), which in turn has been shown to make you more prone to certain medical conditions. People with a larger waist measurement have a higher risk of diabetes and heart disease.

Here's the low-down. You're in the 'watch-out' category if:

- You're a man whose waist measures more than 94 cm (37 in).
- You're a woman whose waist measures more than 80 cm (32 in).
- You're a man of South Asian origin (such men have been found to be even more at risk) whose waist measures more than 90 cm (36 in).

So, getting closer to a pear-shape may actually offer some protection. This is where GiP can help. Choosing foods that are low in points and keeping to the right number of daily points for you, on average, while taking on board the physical activity guidelines (see Chapter 11) can help to reduce excess abdominal fat, getting you into that ideal body shape. And when you reach your target, phase three (Keep-it) is just the ticket for staying in shape – forever.

Take the sticky tape test

Find an old belt and use some brightly coloured sticky tape to mark the section that fits you today. As your waist/belly gets smaller in the coming weeks and months, add more pieces of tape so you can see how well you're doing. Keep the belt for old time's sake – you might need something to prove to your friends what your waist used to look like!

Keeping the weight off

Get to the stage where you want to keep to your healthier eating habits and activity levels, because the pay-off encourages you to carry on. It's all about motivation. You want to stay there because you recognise that the results are greater than they would be if you went back to your old ways. Think about how you got to your target weight and all the benefits this has given you. Write them down and look at your list often. If you have reached your target weight sensibly you won't just have been eating less, you will have changed your shopping and cooking habits too. So set yourself small targets to keep yourself motivated.

Stay slim tips:

- Your Keep-it GiP diet is your new way of life. You may lapse occasionally, that's fine. Just acknowledge it and start again.
- If you put on a pound or two you can always take it off again, so don't punish yourself. Just get back on track.
- Find ways to make your work routine and your family support you. You are going to *stay* slim and healthy.
- Before you reach for the biscuit barrel, ask yourself if it's going to take you nearer to the 'new' you. If it isn't, walk to the fruit bowl!
- Stay fit with family and friends. It's much more fun

to go cycling or swimming or play sport with other people.

● Keep a daily food and mood diary (page 332) so you can see when you indulge and what your emotions are like at that time, for example, boredom, stress, comfort, security, PMT.

● Now that you have reached your target, what are you going to do next? Why not learn a new sport, or take up a new hobby? Better still, as you start your goal, take up a new interest so that your mind has something to occupy itself.

● Treat yourself to some new clothes. Turn out your wardrobe and donate your over-sized clothes to charity. If you make an effort to look good, you'll want to stay slim.

● Be specific about your goal. On that date (specify) I will weigh X.

● Each morning, pour your daily allowance of milk (200 ml/⅓ pint) into a bottle or container. It's an easy way to keep track of your milk. Cereals in the Point Table already have milk included.

Getting started

How do I get started? You can start right here, right now!

1 Weigh yourself. And weigh yourself weekly on the same day, wearing similar clothing.

2 Look at the BMI chart to find your target weight.

3 Measure your waist and work out if you are an 'apple' or 'pear' shape so you know where you want to be heading.

4 Come on board the Start-it Phase using the suggested number of GiPs for your sex.

5 Optional (but strongly advised): Do the exercise on imagining the new you (see page 4).

6 Stock up on some low-GiP foods using our Smart Shopping tips (see Chapter 4).

7 Display the GiP rules in a prominent place so you can look at them often.

8 Move on to Lose-it after the first two weeks, starting with the suggested number of GiPs. Gauge your progress at the end of week three and increase the GiPs by 3 points or so to slow down your weight loss if it's more than 1 kg (2 lb) a week.

9 Keep losing it till you reach your target 'happy' weight. Slide into Keep-it, increasing your GiPs without increasing your hips till you are maintaining your new weight.

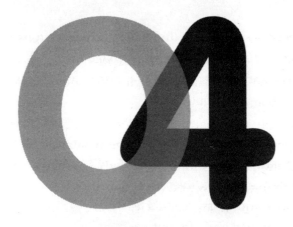

SMART SHOPPING

Walking down the aisle

Whether you're whizzing round the store in 20 minutes, or shopping on the internet, this chapter gives you a speedy low-down on which foods to throw in your trolley. And don't worry if you're hooked on supermarket quick fixes, just check out our Food in a Flash section (page 64).

By now you will know that GiP-eating is about filling and varied goods – not about specialist health food shopping. There are no aisles that need to be avoided. Here's a trick you can play to take home a happy and healthy shopping basket. Imagine your supermarket store is divided into five sections representing the main food groups (page 158).

The largest section is at the top and the smallest section is at the bottom:

- Bread, other cereals, such as breakfast cereals, and potatoes.
- Fruit and vegetables.
- Milk and dairy products.
- Meat, fish and alternatives.
- Fatty and sugary foods.

Your trolley should contain foods roughly in line with these groups of food. You could even try dividing your time in proportion too. For example, spend more time looking at the variety of fruit and vegetables and high-fibre cereals now available and less time on the smaller sections, like the fatty snack foods. This will help you make healthy choices and will also add variety to your diet. You might find that shopping on the internet saves you money because it stops you buying foods from less healthy aisles, as you're not tempted by the smells of the bakery or the buy-one-get-one-free offers (probably a food you weren't going to buy anyway!).

Foods that are high in fibre tend to be low in GiPs. But that's not always the case, because some high-fibre foods may be packed with sugar, or they may simply have a higher glycaemic value than you'd expect (rice cakes have a high GI for example). So, to keep it simple, just glance at the list below so you know what the usual suspects are going to be. You might like to take a photocopy of these pages with you and just highlight what you need that day. You'll soon get to know which foods to grab and which foods to leave for the other shoppers.

Shopping list of low-GiP foods

Here is a selection of foods and drinks – choose the ones you like. They are all low in GiPs.

Drinks
Diet soft drinks
Drinking yoghurt
Juice, grapefruit, unsweetened
Juice, orange, unsweetened
Juice, pineapple, unsweetened
Juice, tomato
Milk, flavoured, pasteurised, chocolate, reduced-fat
Nesquik Chocolate made with semi-skimmed milk
Nesquik Strawberry made with semi-skimmed milk
Soya, non-dairy alternative to milk, unsweetened
Squash, sugar-free
Water, still, sparkling or flavoured

Fresh fruit

Apples

Apricots

Bananas

Cherries

Grapefruit

Grapes

Kiwi fruit

Mangoes

Melon, cantaloupe

Olives

Oranges

Paw-paw

Peaches

Pears

Pineapple

Plums

Strawberries

Canned fruit

Fruit cocktail, in juice

Peaches, in juice

Pears, in juice

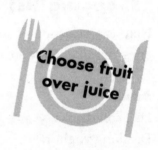

Choose fruit over juice

Dried fruit

Apricots

Dates

Figs

Prunes, ready-to-eat

Raisins

Sultanas

Fresh vegetables

Beetroot

Broccoli

Brussels sprouts

Cabbage

Carrots

Cassava

Cauliflower

Celeriac

Celery

Courgettes

Cucumber

Fennel

Lettuce

Mushrooms

Plantain
Potatoes
Pumpkin
Salad vegetables
Swede

Sweetcorn, baby
Sweetcorn, on-the-cob,
  whole
Sweet potatoes
Yams

Frozen vegetables

Broccoli
Brussels sprouts
Cabbage
Carrots
Cauliflower
French beans

Peas
Runner beans
Spinach
Sweetcorn, baby or
  kernels

Canned vegetables and soups

Ackee
Baked beans
Breadfruit
Chick peas
Chilli beans

Kidney beans
Lentil soup
Peas
Sweetcorn
Tomato soup

Cereals

Bran flakes
High-fibre cereals such as All Bran, muesli
Original porridge oats – large-flake variety
Special K

Avoid temptation
– shop on
the internet

Breads

Barley and sunflower bread
Barley bread*
Burgen oat bran, barley and honey bread*
Burgen soya and linseed bread*
Chapatis, made without fat
Granary bread
Mixed-grain bread
Pumpernickel bread
Rye bread
Wheat tortillas*
White bread, 'with added fibre'

*These foods have lower points compared to the other listed breads.

Bakery

Banana bread
Crumpets
Currant bread or fruit loaf
Currant buns

Dairy chiller cabinet

Fromage frais, virtually fat-free
Ice cream, dairy, reduced calorie
Milk, flavoured, chocolate, reduced-fat
Milk, semi-skimmed
Milk, skimmed
Mousse, reduced-fat

Soya, alternative to yoghurt, fruit
Yoghurt, drinking
Yoghurt, low-fat, plain
Yoghurt, virtually fat-free/diet, plain

Pasta
Fettucini, egg
Linguini, thin or thick
Macaroni
Pasta, plain
Spaghetti, white
Spaghetti, wholemeal

Look for reduced or no added sugar or salt labels

Rice and grains
Barley
Brown rice
Bulgur
Noodles, instant or rice
White rice, Bangladeshi
White rice, basmati
White rice, precooked, microwavable

Dried beans and lentils
Blackeye beans, dried
Black gram, urad gram, dried
Butter beans, dried
Chick peas, split, dried
Chick peas, whole, dried
Haricot beans, dried

Lentils, red, split, dried
Mung beans, whole, dried
Pigeon peas, whole, dried
Pinto beans, dried
Red kidney beans, dried
Soya beans, dried

Miscellaneous
Beetroot, pickled
Gherkins, pickled
Instant noodle soup, packet
Minestrone soup, packet
Quorn (usually chilled or frozen)
Tomato soup, packet
Tzatziki

Other regular shopping-basket items
Eggs
Fish
Flavourings (to taste)
Lean meats and poultry
Oil, olive, rapeseed, spray oil (any)

Healthy shopping tips

● Watch out for ever-increasing portion sizes of
ready meals and snacks such as sandwiches, crisps
and chocolate bars. Just switching from a standard
bag of crisps to a large bag would lead to a weight

gain of over 6 kg (13 lb) over a year without changing anything else!

● Canned foods such as fruit, vegetables, pulses and
fish are a useful purchase. Look for those labelled
reduced, or no added, sugar or salt.

● Dried and frozen foods are often just as nutritious as
fresh, and more convenient if you don't shop often.

● Shop when you've eaten, so it's easier to resist the
temptation to buy high-fat, high-sugar foods. Make
a shopping list and stick to it.

Many supermarkets provide leaflets on healthy eating
and slimming, guiding shoppers to healthy choices.
Some supermarkets even organise 'store tours' run by
local Registered Dietitians. This is a great way to see
your local store in a different light. Consumers find
them informative and enjoyable. Why not ask at
customer services? You may even generate a demand!

You could also look out for a healthy-eating logo,
which all the major supermarkets have. Usually the
products will be lower in fat than the standard item
and may be lower in calories, sugar and salt, too. But
be suspicious of labels boasting 'healthy' desserts and
cakes – they might be lower in fat but higher in sugar.
This could mean they are not necessarily lower in
calories so not a great help if you're weight-watching.
And remember that a reduced-fat version of a high-fat
food isn't a licence to grab and go; it could still pile on
the fat, so don't go eating twice as much.

Food in a flash

Let's face it, who has the time to cook a slap-up meal every night? With today's hectic lifestyles, it's hardly surprising that we get tempted by 'microwave in three minutes' or 'just stir into cooked pasta' labels. And what's wrong with that? Nothing, if you're a wise Gipper. It's all about pick 'n' mix, mix and match. As you know, throwing in a low-GiP food will lower the GI of your meal. The good news about the GiP system is that you can still eat convenience foods, so long as you follow some basic guidelines.

If you know the GiP value of the food, you're well on your way. Just add it to your daily points. If you don't know the GiP value, then:

1 Choose high-fibre versions where possible – many bought foods will be processed, which often makes them lower in fibre than similar products you'd make at home.
2 Choose the right carbs – pitta bread instead of French baguette, basmati rice rather than regular rice, boiled potatoes in their skins instead of instant mash.
3 Go for foods that are as close to their 'whole state' as you can find, such as chunky tomato pasta sauces. Opt for whole-bean soups, and whole vegetables rather than puréed or creamed versions.
4 Mixing and matching really works – throw in a low-GiP food, such as salad, your favourite veg,

Shop wisely!

● Use the shopping list to select those foods that fit in with your Gi Point Diet. Stock up your fridge, larder, freezer and secret snack cupboard with all the goodies that will help you reach your goals.

● See the menu-planning chapter (page 73) for ideas of other foods to buy for the coming week. If, for example, you decide to choose the number 2 meal swap (see page 88), then list the foods that you will need to have at home.

grainy bread or a handful of seeds. Or give your meal a low-GI twist by adding a fruity dessert.

5 Check out the fat and calories against your guideline daily amounts (table on page 66) and watch out for saturated fats. See table on page 70 to find out whether a food has a little or a lot.

What does the label say?

You just need to scan the food packets in your larder to see that we're bombarded by nutritional information, healthy-eating logos and promotional captions. How on earth do we interpret them, and how do we know which labels to trust? If a fromage frais has six per cent fat, is that a lot, or not? Why is reduced-fat cheese called that when, in fact, it's a high-fat food? And did you know that some so-called 'healthy' cereal bars contain as much as 25 per cent sugar?

Here's how to tell your 'low-fats' from your 'fat-frees' and your 'no added sugars' from your 'sugar-frees'.

First, before you interpret the small print, it's helpful to know what you're aiming for. Many food labels now list Guideline Daily Amounts (GDAs). These are guidelines for the average amounts of fats, calories and other nutrients recommended in a healthy adult diet. Obviously, they are only general guidelines, as your personal needs will vary according to your age, weight, physical activity level, and so on.

Nevertheless, GDAs can help you to see whether a particular food might fit into your meals.

Guideline Daily Amounts of nutrients for adults

Nutrient	Men	Women
Calories	2500	2000
Fat	95 g	70 g
Saturated fat	30 g	20 g
Added sugar	30 g	20 g
Salt	7 g	5 g
Fibre	20 g	16 g

So, looking at this, you know the maximum amounts of fat, sugar and so on you need in a day. When you look at the label on a pack of choc-chip cookies, you'll notice that you get around 3 g of fat per cookie. Sounds okay. Add a couple of these to the fat from your cheese and tomato sandwich and packet of crisps, and you've scoffed around 30 g of fat before you've even thought about dinner, or added in what you had for breakfast.

Manufacturers are now starting to use terms on their food labels that have officially recognised meanings. Here's an insight:

Guidelines of common nutrient claims

Nutrition claim	Definition per 100 g or 100 ml	Example
	Contains less than	
Low sugar	5 g sugar	Low-sugar custard
Low-fat	3 g fat	Low-fat rice pudding
Low sodium	40 mg	Low-salt soy sauce
Reduced sugar	Contains 25% less	Reduced-sugar jams
Reduced-fat	sugar, fat or salt	Reduced-fat spreads
Reduced salt	than normal product	Reduced-salt baked beans
Sugar free	Contains less than 0.2 g sugar	Sugar-free jelly Sugar-free squashes Sugar-free fizzy drinks (may be called 'diet')
No added sugar/ unsweetened	No sugars, or foods composed mainly of sugars, have been added to the food	Unsweetened fruit juices

In the past, manufacturers have sometimes added to the confusion by using 'per cent fat-free' claims. Think about it – an '85 per cent fat-free food' still contains a hefty 15 per cent fat! How misleading is that? Nowadays this practice has been more tightly controlled (apart from the quite reasonable '97 per cent fat-free' on some products which only contain three per cent fat).

You may want to study food labels to help you decide how certain foods could fit into your diet, as this helps you to get the most out of the foods you enjoy. This is where reading and understanding the more detailed nutritional information can be a skill worth acquiring. Here's how …

Understanding nutrition information on food labels

The ingredients list will tell you what's in a food but not how much. Ingredients are listed in descending order of weight, so the first ingredient will be present in the largest quantity and the last ingredient will be the smallest. Before we had nutritional information on labels, this was quite useful. But the nutritional content is far more relevant. Even if sugar is near the top of the list it doesn't necessarily mean that food is packed with sugar. It all depends on how much. Remember, sugar does come in different guises, such as sucrose, dextrose, glucose syrup and maltose.

Some manufacturers will display even more detailed nutrition information. This is not yet compulsory on foods unless the manufacturer makes a particular nutrient claim, as shown in the table on page 67. The format is not yet standardised. The table below shows a popular version of nutrition information sometimes referred to as the 'Big Eight'.

Note: energy values are given in kiloJoules (kJ) and kilocalories (kcal). Although not strictly scientifically correct, kilocalories are referred to as 'calories' in everyday speech.

Typical nutrition panel showing the 'Big 8' nutrients

Lentil Soup Typical values	Per 100 g	Per 415 g serving
Energy	190 kJ/45 kcal	795 kJ/190 kcal
Protein	2.6 g	10.8 g
Carbohydrate	6.7 g	27.8 g
– of which sugars	2.6 g	10.8 g
Fat	0.9 g	3.7 g
– of which saturates	0.3 g	1.2 g
Fibre	1.2 g	5.0 g
Sodium*	0.05 g	0.21 g
Equivalent as salt	0.1 g	0.5 g

* Either sodium or salt may be listed (see page 153, Eating for Complete Health)

How do you compare foods?

Nutritional information can help you to decide whether a food has a little or a lot of something. The table below shows guidelines for determining this. When you look at a food label, get into the habit of thinking about how often and how much of that food you would normally eat. A food may be high in fat and/or sugar, but if you only eat small amounts of it occasionally, then that's cool. For these foods use the 'per 100 g' value to see if they contain a little or a lot. This 'per 100 g' value is also useful for comparing two similar products, such as ready-made sauces, to see which is healthier.

For foods that you eat frequently or in large amounts, it's more appropriate to use the nutrition information given 'per serving'. Pick a couple of new foods each week and read the labels so you gradually become aware of suitable convenience foods – there's no need to do the whole trolley all at once.

How to tell if a food contains a little or a lot of a particular ingredient

A lot	A little
10 g of sugars	2 g of sugars
20 g of fat	3 g of fat
5 g of saturates	1 g of saturates
3 g of fibre	0.5 g of fibre
0.5 g of sodium	0.1 g of sodium
1.5 g of salt	0.3 g of salt

Since embracing a new mental approach, here is the difference that it has made to Hazel.

Hazel's testimonial

'I've not had any biscuits, cakes, chocolate and very little ice cream. I feel very different. No longer does the biscuit box cry out to me when I walk past.

'I took my daughters shopping to Tesco's on Monday evening and bought them a cake and a drink while we were there. There were no cries of woe from my stomach or brain and no pangs of jealousy from my heart. I did not care that I wasn't having any. I am now able to say "no thanks" to things for the first time without the niggle of "why not?".

'I have tried quite a lot of the diets around – some with a degree of success – but it always felt wrong. I'm not dieting but eating more healthily and it is not a problem. I even managed a night at the sports club where my daughter goes, without buying a handful of the pick-and-mix I usually have.'

Summary

- It's okay to eat convenience foods, just follow the guidelines.
- Use our shopping list to select foods which dovetail with your Gi Point Diet.
- A food may be high in fat or sugar, but small, occasional amounts is okay!

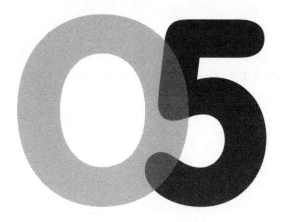

HASTY AND TASTY

MEAL AND MENU IDEAS

There's no such thing as a free lunch or dinner!

Eating the GiP way is like choosing from a Chinese menu – you go for those foods that tempt the taste buds and fit the budget. With GiP eating, you choose a range of tasty treats and make them fit into your

Success is simply a matter of luck. Ask any failure!
(Earl Wilson)

Have you heard the one about the accomplished golfer? A young sporting journalist commented about how lucky she was, to which she replied, 'Yes, funny that. The more I practise, the luckier I get!'

daily points. You'll find that the more you practise GiP eating, the easier it gets. Remember for all these meals to picture your plate (GiP Rule 4, page 42).

Fill up with a low-GI breakfast

Breakfast, just as granny used to say, is the most important meal of the day. It *breaks* the *fast* of night-time (hence the name). It gets your blood glucose up, which leads to a raised level of blood sugar circulating round your brain, helping you to concentrate. And as you know, low-GiP cereals help stabilise blood glucose, helping you to stay alert for that mid-morning meeting – and you're less likely to crave those iced buns. If you can't face a bowl of cereal, try tea and wholegrain toast, a yoghurt smoothie, or some unsweetened fruit juice and a few dried apricots.

Always make time for something at breakfast, even if it is something you grab as you speed out of the door. Think especially about your carbohydrate choices: here are some ideas. Turn also to page 83 for the points values of our breakfast combos.

Choosing your breakfast carbs

Breakfast cereals: Avoid breakfast cereals with a high sugar content. When choosing cereals look for high-fibre cereals such as All Bran. Muesli is a good choice too. Add some of your favourite fruits, a sprinkling of chopped walnuts and natural yoghurt.

Porridge: This is one of the best low-GI breakfast foods ever invented. Instant hot oats are a convenient substitute, though they are higher in GI as they are more processed.

Top Tip: Try making some speedy porridge in the microwave. Check the packet for instructions.

Bread: Toast is always a favourite but choose your bread carefully. Go for grainy varieties such as soy and linseed or multigrain. For variety, why not try toasted fruit loaf?

Top Tip: Tasty toast toppers include beans on oat bran, barley and honey toast with a dash of Worcestershire sauce (4.5 GiPs); grilled lean bacon and sliced tomato on two slices of granary toast (6.5 GiPs); sliced banana on two slices of currant bread (6 GiPs). And for a cook-up, try a plain omelette with grilled field mushrooms (3 GiPs), poached egg on crumpets (5.5 GiPs), or grilled lean bacon, canned plum tomatoes and scrambled eggs (6.5 GiPs).

Milk and juices: If you've bolted out the door without even thinking about food, you could pick up a drinking yoghurt or an individual carton of milk on your way to work. Look out for lower-fat milkshakes, or make yourself a chocolate shake at work.

Top Tip: Got time? Why not make a smoothie – blend together your favourite fruit (fresh or canned) with skimmed or semi-skimmed milk and yoghurt.

Fill up with a low-GI lunch

Your low-GI breakfast and mid-morning snack will keep your energy levels raised throughout the morning. That mid-morning snack not only keeps blood glucose stable, it also prevents you from overeating at lunchtime. And the effect of a low GI breakfast and mid-morning snack will last you till lunchtime. By lunchtime, it's time to refuel with a right carbs lunch.

● Make or buy sandwiches made with suitable bread and low-fat fillings such as lean meat, chicken or fish with plenty of salad. Avoid mayonnaise, as it is high in fat. Instead, choose mustard, pickles, chutney, salsa or lemon juice to add flavour.

● Create your own salad using a variety of salad vegetables, add canned mixed beans (count as 2 GiPs), tuna (1 GiP), mozzarella cheese (3 GiPs) or egg (2 GiPs). Avoid oil-based salad dressings. For a real zing, why not try hot sauce, lemon juice and black pepper?

- Make your own pasta salad: boil your favourite pasta, add some chopped ham, tuna or reduced-fat cheese. Toss in some extra beans and salad vegetables and mix together with low-fat natural yoghurt and herbs for a creamy dressing.

- Turn to page 85 for the points values of our lunch combos.

Choosing your lunch and main-meal carbs

Bread: Choose grainy, dense breads with whole seeds for your sandwiches or with your main meal. Multigrain, granary, soya and linseed, rye, 100 per cent stoneground wholemeal, oatbran and barley breads are all good choices.

Potatoes: Most potatoes have a high GI, new potatoes are slightly lower. They are, however, a nutritious part of the diet, so rather than cutting them out make sure you include other low-GI carbohydrates with them. Alternatively, why not try sweet potatoes, which have a low GI and taste delicious when baked or microwaved.

Pasta: Enjoy with your lunch-time salad or as your main meal. Most pasta has a low GI. Cook until *al dente* and remember, watch what you serve pasta with – avoid creamy high-calorie sauces.

Rice: Choose basmati rice, long-grain or brown rice. For an alternative to pasta or rice, bulgur wheat (cracked wheat) has a low GI and tastes great in salads.

Beans and pulses: As well as being low-GI foods, beans and pulses are a great source of protein, iron and fibre. Include them in your meals wherever possible – have stir-fried beans, beany casseroles and soups, or just chuck them into any salad; they will help lower the GI of the meal.

Vegetables and salad: Great for lowering the GI of a meal and full of important antioxidant vitamins and minerals. Vegetables and salad should always feature

Eat these...	Instead of ...
Muesli, porridge, bran cereals	Cornflakes, puffed wheat
Grainy bread, such as soft-grain white or multi-grain	White or wholemeal bread
Unsweetened fruit juice, diet drink or water	Sugared fizzy drinks
Boiled new potatoes in their skin, or sweet potato	French fries or mashed potato
Lean meat, poultry without the skin, fish	Fatty meat
Currant bun or small muffin	Danish pastry or doughnut
Lentil-based dishes	Meat-based dishes
Oatmeal biscuits	Wheatmeal biscuits

in your lunch-time and main meals. Fresh, frozen and canned all count towards your five-a-day recommended intake – the more variety and colour the better.

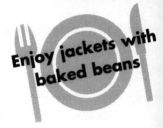

Enjoy jackets with baked beans

Dinner time!

Having a dinner dilemma? Want something quick and easy to prepare after a hard day at work? Or do you want to impress friends or family but still stick to your low-GI diet? There are four important points to consider to ensure your meal is healthy and well balanced:

- Base your meal on a low-GI carbohydrate – pasta, noodles, sweet potato, grains such as bulgur wheat or barley, basmati rice, new potatoes, beans and pulses.
- Make sure you include generous amounts of vegetables or salad, or ideally both!
- Always include some protein such as lean meat, poultry, fish, eggs, reduced-fat cheese, beans and pulses, or a handful of nuts. You could use peas, beans, lentils and chickpeas to extend meat dishes. For example, mixing some lentils with a bolognese sauce can make it go further, while lowering the GI.
- Watch the fat. Use healthy cooking methods that require little oil, such as stir-frying, steaming,

poaching and baking. Avoid high-fat sauces and dressings that contain butter, cream or lots of oil. Look for reduced-fat dairy products such as low-fat yoghurt or reduced-fat crème fraîche or cheese.
● For healthy low-carb dinner combos, turn to page 88.

In a jiffy

The same rules apply if you are eating a ready-prepared meal. When choosing a ready meal make sure it contains some low-GI carbohydrate and some lean protein.

Many supermarkets now offer a healthier low-fat range, which can be a good option. These may contain very few vegetables so always add extra or serve with a side salad. And if you don't have a clue of the GiP

Save a GiP or two

Eat this ...	Instead of ...	Save ...
Oatcakes	Rice cakes	3.5 GiPs
Fruit loaf	Waffle	2.5 GiPs
Drinking yoghurt	Fresh cranberry juice	2 GiPs
Tortilla wrap	White bread	2.5 GiPs
Pitta bread	Baguette	4 GiPs
Canned pears	Canned peaches	1 GiP
Dried figs	Dried dates	1 GiP
Basmati rice	Jasmine rice	5 GiPs
New potatoes	French fries	3 GiPs

value, simply choose the types of foods that you know are low-GI and add some GiP-free goodies.

Desserts

Fortunately many desserts are based on fruit and dairy products, both having a low GI. Fruit cocktail with ice cream carries 3.5 points and a carton of diet yoghurt offers one virtuous Gi Point.

Vegetarian-style eating

Many vegetarian foods have a low GI. It's the way you cook them and what you mix with them that counts:

- Keep your foods as whole as possible.
- Remember that beans and lentils are especially low-GI foods.
- Many fruits also have a low GI. Examples are apples, cherries, grapefruit, pears, strawberries and plums. Peaches and pears canned in juice are also great choices.
- Red lentils, haricot beans, French beans and runner beans have an exceptionally low GI.
- Go easy on the cheese. It contains around 30 per cent fat, mostly saturated. Grate it to go further or choose reduced-fat versions.
- Don't be fooled into thinking that all foods bought from a health food shop are good for you. Many

can be high in fat and sugar, and even though they may be made with wholemeal flour, they are not necessarily healthy.

● Bangladeshi rice is the lowest-GI rice.

Meal swaps

These 'Meal Swaps' or 'Combos' contain calculated meal choices for breakfast, lunch and dinner. You can swap them around on different days. They are your choices for lazy days, when you don't want to think too much about what to eat. You can also plan your shopping around them. In fact, there are 12 different swaps for each meal occasion so you could just do one mad shopping day and you're sorted for almost a fortnight.

Pick and choose from this buffet of delights – opt for the meals that fit in with your points. You'll soon know which ones are your regular 'must-haves'. For in-between-meal goodies, choose from the snacks below or refer to Snack Attack (page 99).

Remember GiP Rule 1 – Eat three meals and three snacks every day.

These swaps are filling and balanced meal choices. If you're looking for a meal with lower points, feel free to leave out some items, or have them later as one of your snacks.

Combo Breakfast Choices	Portion size	GiPs
1 All Bran and semi-skimmed milk	5 tbsp+200 ml (⅓ pint)	2
1 small banana		2
		4
2 Branflakes and semi-skimmed milk	4 tbsp+200 ml (⅓ pint)	4
1 fresh apple		0.5
		4.5
3 Porridge, made with milk and water	6 tbsp of made-up porridge using 100 ml (¼ pint) milk and water as required	3.5
Honey	1 teaspoon	1
Tomato juice	1 glass (150 ml)	0
		4.5
4 Muesli and semi-skimmed milk	3 tbsp+200 ml (⅓ pint)	4
Pineapple juice, unsweetened	1 glass (150 ml)	1.5
		5.5

Eat basmati rice instead of jasmine

Combo Breakfast Choices	Portion size	GiPs
5 Special K and semi-skimmed milk	5 tbsp+200 ml (⅓ pint)	4
Fresh grapefruit		0
		4
6 Bran Flakes and semi-skimmed milk	4 tbsp+200 ml (⅓ pint)	4
Poached eggs	2	1.5
		5.5
7 Instant hot oats made with semi-skimmed milk	follow pack instructions using 200 ml (⅓ pint) milk	4.5
1 fresh pear		0.5
		5
8 Weetabix and semi-skimmed milk	2 biscuits+200 ml (⅓ pint)	4.5
Tomato juice	1 glass (150 ml)	0
		4.5
9 Peanut butter on 1 slice of wholemeal bread	2 tsp peanut butter	3.5
Canteloupe melon	½ melon	2
		5.5

Combo Breakfast Choices	GiPs
10 Wholemeal bread (2 slices) with low-fat spread and banana (1)	6
11 Granary bread (2 slices) with scrambled egg (2) and tomato	6
12 Wholemeal bread (2 slices) with butter (1 tsp) and poached eggs (2)	8

Combo Lunch Choices with Dessert	GiPs
1 Burgen soya and linseed bread (2 slices) with low-fat spread (1 tsp), tuna (small can) and cucumber	3
Reduced-fat chocolate mousse	1.5
	4.5
2 Wheat tortilla (1) with chicken (3 slices) and mixed green salad	4
Diet yoghurt	1
	5
3 Wheat tortilla (1) with mozzarella cheese (small matchbox-size piece, chopped), beef tomato and basil	4.5
Grapes (15)	2
	6.5

Combo Lunch Choices with Dessert	GiPs
4 Granary bread (2 slices) with low-fat spread (1 tsp), ham (2 slices) and salad	5
Olives (10)	0.5
	5.5
5 Granary bread (2 slices) with low-fat spread (1 tsp), mozzarella cheese (1 slice), fresh basil and tomato	5.5
Apple	0.5
	6
6 Pumpernickel bread (2 slices) and low-fat spread (1 tsp), ham (2 slices), mixed green salad	5.5
Chocolate flavoured milk, reduced-fat (200 ml (⅓ pint))	1
	6.5
7 Jacket potato with low-fat spread (1 tsp), cottage cheese (small tub) and sliced peppers	6.5
Plums (3)	0.5
	7

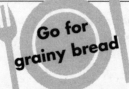

Go for grainy bread

Combo Lunch Choices with Dessert	GiPs
8 Wholemeal bread (2 slices) with low-fat spread (1 tsp), cottage cheese (small tub) and shredded cucumber and lettuce	6.5
Fromage frais, virtually fat-free (small pot)	1.5
	8
9 Jacket potato with low-fat spread (1 tsp), tuna (small can) and sweetcorn (3 tablespoons)	7
Packet minestrone soup	0
	7
10 Wholemeal bread (2 slices) with low-fat spread (1 tsp), melted Edam (1 slice) and tomato	7
Canned peaches, in juices (6 slices) with sugar-free jelly	0.5
	7.5
11 Jacket potato with low-fat spread (1 tsp), half-fat cheddar cheese (3 tablespoons grated) and side salad (fat-free dressing)	9.5
Fresh strawberries (teacupful)	0
	9.5
12 Baguette (1 small) with low-fat spread (1 tsp), prawns (small jar) and mixed green salad (fat-free dressing)	10.5
Fresh pear	0.5
	11

Main Meal Choices	Portion size	GiPs
1 Garlic Mushrooms		0
Cod Kebabs with Fresh Dill		1.5
Mixed salad		0
Tortilla wrap		3
		4.5
2 Sizzling Turkey Burgers		1.5
Hamburger bun		5
Chilli and Lime Rocket Leaves		0
Fruit cocktail in natural juice ½ can		1
		7.5
3 Turkey Stroganoff		1.5
Basmati rice	2 serving spoons*	2.5
Grilled tomato salad		0
Orange juice, unsweetened	150 ml glass	1.5
		5.5
4 Herby Pork Chops		2
Boiled potatoes	3 egg-sized	3
Steamed spinach		0
Steamed turnips		0
Fresh apple		0.5
		5.5

* 1 serving spoon = 3 tablespoons

(Recipes for all of these meals are in Chapter 8.)

Main Meal Choices	Portion size	GiPs
5 Haddock with Thai Green Pepper and Basil Sauce		2.5
Instant noodles	5 tablespoons	2
Side salad in fat-free dressing		0
Sugar-free jelly and whole strawberries		0
		4.5
6 Baked Tiger Prawns		1
Cheesy Pork Chops		2.5
New potatoes, boiled	4	3
Grilled aubergine		0
Pickled onions		0
		6.5
7 Sweet and Sour Chicken Drumsticks		3
Middle Eastern Tabouleh Salad		3
Kiwi fruit	2	1.5
		7.5
8 Salmon Steaks in Garlicky Balsamic Vinegar		3.5
Boiled egg fettucine	5 tablespoons	1.5
Steamed asparagus tips		0
Peaches, canned in juice	6 slices	0.5
		5.5

Main Meal Choices	Portion size	GiPs
9 Couscous with Peppers and Red Onion		4.5
Chilli beans	½ large can	1
Lettuce, cucumber, tomato, red onion salad		0
		5.5
10 Warming Marrow and Leek Soup		0
Mediterranean Pasta		5
Green herby salad (watercress, mixed lettuce leaves, fresh herbs, lime juice, black pepper)		0
Low-fat natural yoghurt		1
Fresh cherries	12 cherries	0.5
		6.5
11 Instant Noodles with Prawns and Garlic		6.5
Herby Baby Spinach and Beansprouts		0
Peaches, canned in juice	6 slices	0.5
		7
12 Beef Chow Mein		7
Stir-fried Babycorn		0
Tomato juice	150 ml glass	0
		7

Starters and Sides*	GiPs
Al Dente Asparagus	0
Balsamic French Beans	0
Beef Tomatoes with Black Olives	1
Cabbage with Fennel Seeds	0
Char-grilled Vegetables with Honey and Basil	2
Chilli and Honey Chicken Wings	2
Chilli and Lime Rocket Leaves	0
Chilli Peanut Popcorn	2.5
Courgette Boats	0
Cucumber and Mint Cooler	0
Curried Cauliflower	1
Curried Okra	0
Garlic Mushrooms	0
Gherkin and Onion Pickle	0
Grilled Tomato Salad	0
Herby Baby Spinach and Beansprouts	0
Hot Roasted Vegetables	0
Jelly with Whole Strawberries	0
Layered Mushroom and Tomato with Grilled Cheese	1
Savoy Cabbage with Caraway Seeds	0
Speedy Salsa Sauce	0
Spiced Vegetables	0
Stir-fried Babycorn	0
Warming Marrow and Leek Soup	0
Wheat-free Tabouleh	0

* these dishes can also be used as snacks

Grab-a-snack	Portion size	GiPs
Cereal chewy bar – dried fruit	45–50 g bar	4.5
Cereal crunchy bar – dried fruit	45–50 g bar	4.5
Fromage frais, virtually fat-free	1 pot	1.5
Milk:		
Chocolate flavoured, reduced-fat	200 ml	1
Strawberry Nesquik made with semi-skimmed milk	200 ml	1
Nuts*:		
Almonds	10–12	3
Cashews	15	3.5
Peanuts, dry roasted	25 g/1 oz	3
Peanuts, roasted and salted	25 g/1 oz	3
Walnuts	6 halves	3
Popcorn, plain	5 tablespoons	4
Soup:		
Minestrone, dried, as served	1 soup bowl	0
Tomato, dried, as served	1 soup bowl	0.5
Yoghurt:		
Diet	small pot	1
Low-fat, natural	small pot	1

* strictly once a day

Sample menus

Below are five sample menu plans from real dieters. The 17- and 20-point plans are from women, and the 22- and 25-point plans are from men. There's also a vegetarian one that you can enjoy if this is your preference. These quick and easy menus will inspire you with many more ideas and show you it's simple to put the diet into practice. You might like to jot down your own plans so that you can reuse them to save you time. Visit www.gipointdiet.com for more ideas.

17-point sample menu, Start-it Phase

Breakfast:	All Bran with semi-skimmed milk	2.5
	Fresh pear	0.5
Snack:	Chewy cereal bar	4.5
Lunch:	Garlic and tomato herb fettucine	
	(requested no oil when out to lunch)	
	5 tablespoons fettucine	1.5
	Tomatoes, onions, herbs, garlic	0
	Mixed free salad, no dressing	0
Snack:	Apple	0.5
Dinner:	Spiced lemon sole with potatoes and vegetables	
	Lemon sole, grilled	1
	Broccoli, steamed	0
	Baby corn	0
	Carrots, 2 serving spoons	1
	Potatoes, boiled	3

	Chilli sauce, salt/pepper	0
Fruit:	8 prunes	1.5
Night snack:	Diet yoghurt	1
Unlimited still water		0
Total		**17**

Additional free daily allowance:

	200 ml (⅓ pint) semi-skimmed milk	0.5

20-point sample menu, Lose-it Phase

Breakfast:	Reduced-sugar muesli with semi-skimmed milk	4
Snack:	Fun-size Snickers bar	2
Lunch:	Home-made weekend veggie rice	
	Basmati rice	2.5
	Kidney beans (canned)	2
	Tomatoes (canned)	0
	Onions, herbs and spices	0
Snack:	Low-fat natural yoghurt	1
Dinner:	Chilli chicken with sweet potato and salad	
	Chicken breast	2
	Baked sweet potato	3
	Broccoli, steamed	0
	Chilli sauce	0
	Large side salad (celery, tomato, cucumber, lettuce, red onion)	0

Night snack:	Peanut butter on a slice of wholemeal toast	3.5
Unlimited still water		0
Total		**20**

Additional free daily allowance:

	200 ml (⅓ pint) semi-skimmed milk	0.5

22-point sample menu, Start-it Phase

Breakfast:	Porridge, made with milk and water	3.5
	Tomato juice with Worcester sauce	0
Snack:	Banana	2
Lunch:	Granary bread (toasted)	3.5
	Baked beans, canned in tomato sauce	2
Snack:	15 grapes	2
Dinner:	Roast chicken with new potatoes, carrots, peas and gravy	
	3 slices roast chicken	2
	4 boiled new potatoes	3
	3 tablespoons peas	2
	GiP-free stir-fried baby corn	0
	Instant gravy	0.5
Snack:	Reduced-fat chocolate mousse	1.5
Total		**22**

Additional free daily allowance:

	200 ml (⅓ pint) semi-skimmed milk	0.5
	½ pint of beer from alcohol allowance	

25-point sample menu, Lose-it Phase

Breakfast:	Weetabix and semi-skimmed milk	4.5
Snack:	10 almonds	3
Lunch:	Lentil soup	2
	Granary bread, 2 slices	3.5
Snack:	Orange	1.5
Dinner:	Grilled steak with chips, mushrooms and side salad	
	150 g (5 oz) rump steak, lean, grilled	2
	Chips, 2 serving spoons	
	5 per cent fat, frozen, oven baked	5
	Mushrooms, stir-fried in a little oil	2
	Mixed 'free' salad vegetables	0
Snack:	Pears, canned in juice	1.5
Total		**25**

Additional free daily allowance:

	200 ml (⅓ pint) semi-skimmed milk	0.5

25-point sample menu, vegetarian

Breakfast:	2 slices barley bread	3
	Low-fat spread, scraping	0.5
	1 banana, sliced	2
Snack:	3 plums	0.5
	1 pear	0.5
Lunch:	2 slices white bread	5.5
	Low-fat spread, scraping	0.5
	30 g (1 oz) Edam cheese	2.5

	Tomato	0
	1 apple	0.5
Snack:	6 walnut halves	3
Dinner:	Lentil and vegetable casserole	
	Lentils, cupful of cooked (50 g/2 oz	1
	raw dried) baked in oven with	
	mixed vegetables, tinned tomatoes	
	and vegetable stock, serve with	
	brown rice, 2 serving spoons	2.5
	1 diet yoghurt	1
Snack:	½ cantaloupe melon	2

Total   **25**

Additional free daily allowance:

     200 ml (⅓ pint) semi-skimmed milk   0.5

Summary

- Link pleasure to your meal and menu planning and reach your happy weight in a safe and sustainable way.
- See your plate with two veg portions (v, v), plus one protein (p) and low-GI carb (c): veggie, veggie, protein, carbs!
- Think of your meal as two veg plus meat, and it'll help you keep your portions in perspective.

06

SNACK ATTACK

No time for breakfast ... rushing for the train ... quick snack on the way home. Sound familiar? With our hectic lifestyles today, eating on the run is becoming more common, and so keeping an eye on the fats and figures can be difficult. What's more, fast snacky food isn't necessarily healthy food, and often convenience overrides health. So, how can GiP overcome the snacking blips? What thoughts will influence your choices?

Choices and consequences

When it comes to making a choice, for example, between that iced bun or an apple, which one will you choose? Hmmm – tough choice, eh? Okay, so we all like to indulge from time to time and, on occasion, that's cool. What you might like to think about, though, is that the choices you make today shape your future tomorrow, both physically, in terms of your future health, and mentally, because they affect your overall sense of well-being. Eating that bun today can have an effect on your health, your waistline, and how you feel about yourself once the short-term pleasure it gave you is over.

Healthy snacks can be good for you, however. For example, they're helpful in keeping you alert in the middle of the day. With GI eating, snacks can be your best friends as they help you to keep your blood sugar levels steady. What's more, they can positively help you watch that waistline, since a feeling of fullness means you're less likely to raid the fridge as soon as you drop your briefcase in the hallway.

Having a snack attack?

Here's the low-down on some well-known favourites. How do your choices measure up?

Crudités and dips: A crunchy way to get your anti-oxidants. Fill up on the following to reduce the likelihood of overdoing the calories later. Carrot sticks, cucumber, celery and other crudité veggies are low in GiPs. Opt for healthy dips such as those based on low-fat yoghurt for calcium (such as raita or tzatziki) or tomatoes for lycopene (such as salsa).

Spice up your chick peas: Chick peas are a great source of fibre and protein. Add some fresh lime juice, chilli and chopped coriander leaves. Toss them on to a bed of mixed red onion and watercress salad and you have a substantial snack for only 2½ points. (If you boil them from dried, it comes to only 1½ points.)

Peanuts: Nuts can help to fill you up so that you are less likely to overeat. They contain healthy mono-unsaturated fats and a range of vitamins and minerals. Scientific research suggests that 30 g (1 oz) of peanuts daily may suppress hunger and so promote weight loss, lower blood cholesterol levels, and reduce the risk of type 2 diabetes in women. There is also extensive research on almonds and walnuts. That's why certain nuts are encouraged in the GiP diet once a day. Unsalted nuts are best.

Rice cakes: These are low in calories, yes, but high in GI. Consequently, rice cakes have a high GiP value. Swap two rice cakes for two oatmeal biscuits and you halve the GiPs you spend.

Ice cream: Go for lower-fat versions. Add some sugar-free jelly and fresh whole strawberries for no extra points.

Olives: Satisfying, moist (so you're less likely to wash them down with too much alcohol than you would with a dry salty snack) and rich in healthy monounsaturated fat. Very low in points; keep to recommended portions. Taste not waist!

Popcorn: A healthy snack, high in fibre and protein, but higher in GiPs than sweetcorn, because of the way it changes form when cooked. Make it yourself with a couple of tablespoons of popping corn and a teaspoon of oil, cover and watch 'em pop! Or try Chilli Peanut Popcorn (recipe page 137) which lowers the GiPs by mixing the corn with peanuts.

Snacks in the office
Here are some handy low GiP carbs that you can take to the office. If a healthy snack is accessible, it'll be easier for you to keep to your GiP rules.

- Drinking yoghurt
- Flavoured reduced-fat milk
- Milkshake powder and skimmed or semi-skimmed milk
- Fresh fruit
- Individual canned fruit in juice
- Dried fruit
- Fruit loaf slices
- Currant bun
- Low-fat or diet yoghurt

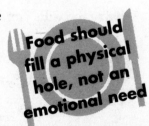
Food should fill a physical hole, not an emotional need

Eat ...	Instead of ...
Oatcakes	Rice cakes
Fun-size Snickers bar	Milk chocolate bar
Half a dozen walnut halves	Pretzels
Cream crackers	Water biscuits
Olives	Cheese chunks
Tzatziki dip made from low-fat yoghurt	Sour cream dip

- Virtually fat-free fromage frais
- 25 g nuts
- Packet soup

GiP-free snacks

Get creative and conjure up a delectable free snack in seconds by using our quick and easy recipes (page 151). Here's the low-down:

Garlic Mushrooms

Cabbage with Fennel Seeds

Grilled Tomato Salad

Courgette Boats

Chilli and Lime Rocket Leaves

Warming Marrow and Leek Soup

Savoy Cabbage with Caraway Seeds

Herby Baby Spinach and Beansprouts

Gherkin and Onion Pickle

Stir-fried Baby Corn

Tasty, filling, low-carb snacks are all part of the plan

Curried Okra
Balsamic French Beans
Hot Roasted Vegetables
Speedy Salsa Sauce
Cucumber and Mint Cooler
Spiced Vegetables
Al Dente Asparagus
Wheat-free Tabouleh
Jelly with Whole Strawberries

Cook-a-snack

Work out your GiPs from the raw ingredients for these substantial snacks or light meals:

- Cheat's pizza – take a slice of pitta bread, smother it in tomato purée and add masses of veggies, such as green peppers, mushrooms, courgettes and tomatoes. Top with a bit of grated cheese, ideally Edam, and a few halved olives.

- Boil up some pasta and throw in some canned tuna, fresh basil, garlic and some cubed reduced-fat feta cheese.

- Southern sweet potato chips – peel and cut a sweet potato into chips. Boil till just cooked. Drizzle over a little olive oil and flavour with Cajun seasoning, black pepper and a touch of lemon juice. Grill or bake.

- Baked courgettes – cut a courgette lengthwise and bake or microwave with coarse black pepper, balsamic vinegar and some spray oil. Smother with toasted sesame seeds.

And a couple of chilled snacks …

- Crudités – chop up your favourite raw veggies and serve with raita (natural low-fat yoghurt mixed with grated cucumber and cumin seeds).
- Banana and peach smoothie – in a blender, whiz up some low-fat fruit yoghurt with a banana and some drained canned peaches.

The comfort cushion

Food should only fill a physical hole, not an emotional need. If you become more aware of the underlying feeling that is causing you to overeat, you are more able to make some changes. You can regain control and experiment with new and healthier ways to satisfy this same need.

You may wish to keep a daily food journal (see page 332) that will highlight the emotional need that causes you to reach for certain snacks. For example, it may arise from boredom, stress, a need for comfort,

I haven't failed. I've just found 10,000 ways that won't work!

security or any other challenging feelings that you are striving to manage. Remind yourself, 'What would have to happen, that is within *my* control, for this need to be met in a healthy and functional way?' Before you seek solace in that 'naughty but nice food', ask yourself whether this is taking you nearer to the 'new' you. If it isn't, choose again! For example, if you find that meditation is as comforting as unhealthy snacking, meditate instead!

Other than changing your dietary choices, you might also consider doing something that you've been promising yourself forever. Maybe take those singing lessons that you've always wanted to do, try a new sport, go salsa dancing, do charity work, take up studying and learn something new that would bring you joy and satisfaction, or develop more meaningful relationships.

Distraction works effectively! Make a creative list of all the things that would work for you, such as going for a walk, having a bath or dancing to your favourite CD. By the time you've done this, your brain will have been tricked into believing that it no longer needs that 'fix'! Treat your healthy food plan as a new way of life. If you lapse occasionally, just acknowledge it and start again.

The key to long-term good snacking is to have a healthy relationship with all types of food. Food has emotional, psychological and social aspects and so it pays to examine your attitude towards food, aiming to get the right balance, most of the time. As soon as you say to yourself that you must avoid a food, what happens? That food becomes even more desirable. Challenge your thinking and attitudes towards food. Get into the habit of knowing which are the low-GiP foods and opt for these, often. And remember that high-GiP foods aren't bad foods – there's a place for all types. You will soon find that you automatically know which of your daily foods are lower and which are a little higher in points. With this knowledge, you can include a healthy mix of foods with confidence.

Are you a Real Gipper?

Question:

Are you a snack-o-holic? If so, when are you likely to indulge?

Choice 1: I go for snacks when I feel hungry, but it's usually fruit, some veggies I keep in a box in the fridge, a cereal bar or a few cashews.

Fab! You are conscious of when you're eating and you are making healthy choices.

Choice 2: When I'm on the go, I'll attack the closest sweet shop or petrol station and look for a sugar fix.

Your blood sugar is more likely to fluctuate from high to low if you graze on sweet stuff. Not such a good idea for Gippers.

Choice 3: When I'm feeling down in the dumps, or a tad under the weather, I could eat all day …

Consequently, your meals and snacks may be less regular, leading you to perhaps making unhealthy food choices. You may be more likely to pile on the pounds as you're less conscious of what you're eating.

Results:

Choice 1: You'll appreciate the high energy and an overall feel-good state, which also means the likelihood of a positive frame of mind.

Choice 2: Choose more filling options like a light wholegrain sandwich, a small pub-sized packet of nuts or a banana. Give yourself an extra boost of motivation and think about the end goal – what it is that you really want, and direct your thoughts in that direction only!

Choice 3: Today's choices become tomorrow's consequences and that includes how you are choosing to feel. Think about supporting someone, in some small way. This way, you'll relieve yourself of the burden of self-obsession! By focusing on others, you'll feel uplifted and are therefore more likely to get back on track with your own goals.

So be a Real Gipper – and choose in line with the new you.

Summary

- Snacks can be good for your mental performance and they help keep blood-glucose levels steady. With GiP eating, low-GI snacks can be your best friends.
- Keep a daily food and mood diary so you can see what makes you over-indulge.
- Get into the habit of knowing the low-GiP snacks – maybe keep them handy at work and make them a regular item on your shopping list.
- Distract yourself. Make a creative and fun list of all the things that would work for you.
- Treat your new healthy food choices as a fresh way of life. If you lapse occasionally, just acknowledge it and start again.

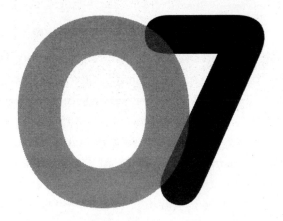

EATING OUT
THE GiP WAY

Your body is a temple ...

And sometimes it's a nightclub! A little of what you fancy does you good, but too much can bring about a different set of consequences, including your weight.

Eating out is one of the pleasures of life, and when you're slimming, there's no reason why you can't join in the fun. Whether it's a business meeting over lunch, dinner with friends or family, or a fast-food take-away when you're on the move, eating out is a part of our lives that's here to stay. And it can be part of your new healthier GI lifestyle.

Pain versus pleasure

Even if you don't know the GiP value of your indulgence, by following our simple tips you can make healthy choices, as well as choosing lower-GI options. More and more restaurants and fast-food outlets are taking notice of the increasing demand for healthier menus. Remember, in a restaurant *you* are the customer and can request changes in the way food is cooked and served. Simply ask. You're paying for it! Here are some tips on eating out to help you on your way.

For starters, no need to advertise that you're 'on a diet'. Your friends will probably start saying, 'Oh, you can just have one today', and you might give in to temptation. Instead, hold your head up high and order these delicious choices with confidence, as GiP-eating isn't about dieting, it's about balance. When you don't tell yourself you're 'on a diet', the rest of the gang will want to know the secrets of your successful weight loss.

Avoid going to a restaurant ravenous for the next mouthful. Instead, grab a piece of fruit or GiP-free food on the way. And get into the habit of putting your fork and knife down after every mouthful; it's amazing how much longer your meal will last.

Remember that you're there to enjoy yourself, so long as this isn't something you do five days a week! Make a mental note of what you've chosen so you can keep track of your points and make up for it at other times if you have overdone it.

Feedback is the currency of life

Your body is the best feedback mechanism available. There will be negative feelings that you link to when you overeat, have one pint too many, or smoke too much. Remember how your head feels? How your mouth

Have a low-GI snack before you visit the take-away joint

resembles the bottom of a parrot's cage? Or the effects on your digestive system of that spicy curry? You might have felt bloated, had a distended tum, or needed to slouch in the armchair with no energy, nursing the mother of all hangovers, with the words 'Never again!' ringing in your ears.

As you sit in the restaurant or queue for the burger, think about these feelings so that you'll start making wise choices. Link more and more pleasurable feelings to your new choices, knowing that they are taking you nearer to the 'new' you. Think about your increased energy levels, the boost in confidence and self-esteem you are getting, and all the other benefits as you get nearer to that ideal, happy weight. Next time you're eating out, perhaps you'll be in the much-dreamt-about little black number!

Ultimately your actions are driven by your deepest desire or intention.

In the restaurant ...

This very week, when you've finally made the decision to start your new healthy living plan, guess what? You're inundated with dinner and party offers! This will test just how committed you really are. Get through this and you've shown what you're made of. No need to join the 'Billy No Mates' club! The first step is to overcome your habit of ordering the richest, most indulgent food on the menu. You'll need some focus and determination to succeed – but succeed you can.

All patterns can be broken. Anything learnt can be unlearnt. Enjoy and continue to draw on the essential tools offered in this book to support you in making the life that you really want. Tell yourself 'I always choose healthily' and look for ways to support this. Here's how you can begin to make those changes by choosing wisely when you're eating out.

Eating Italian

Italian food is not just pizza and pasta: many menus feature grilled meats, chicken and seafood dishes served with plenty of fresh vegetables, all of which can be healthier choices. Here are some GiP tips:

● Most pasta has a low GI, but the sauces served with it can be laden with fat and calories. Order pasta with a fresh tomato sauce, which tends to be lower in fat than cream-based sauces, and say 'no' to the

Parmesan cheese. Ask for your plate to be half filled with a crunchy selection of mixed salad leaves and the other half filled with the pasta of your choice.

- Go for a thin-base pizza with masses of low-GI vegetable toppings. Steer clear of extra cheese and processed pepperoni.

- Ask for a GiP-free salad with your meal. For the dressing, opt for balsamic vinegar or a squeeze of lemon juice and a sprinkling of herbs.

- If you are having a grilled meat or chicken dish, ask for the sauce 'on the side' so you have control over how much you eat, or go without. Ask for unbuttered vegetables and boiled new potatoes in their skins (4 GiPs). Don't be tempted to have the French fries as these have a higher GI and are high in fat (6 GiPs).

- Remember, you may be starving when you're waiting for your meal to arrive but those bread points still count. Rather than garlic bread, choose a healthier low-GI starter such as chunky vegetable soup, melon, Mozzarella and tomato salad or tuna salad with an oil-free dressing.

Eating Indian

If you're ordering group dishes, be careful how much you eat. This is a common pitfall in Indian, Chinese and Thai restaurants. Give yourself a full plate at the beginning of a meal, eat slowly and stop when you've finished. Indian cuisine can be GiP-friendly. Just avoid the high-fat fried foods and heavy, butter-based sauces.

- For the main course, go for a dahl dish, which is made from lentils. There are many different types to choose from. Ask the waiter which dahls are less puréed and choose those – they have a lower Glycaemic Index. For calculating your GiPs, use the cooked dahl value (a cupful has only 3.5 GiPs).
- Opt for chicken, prawn or vegetable dishes, rather than lamb or beef, which tend to be higher in fat. You might see a layer of orange oil on the top – scoop your serving from underneath.
- Go for tandoori chicken or chicken tikka as they are cooked quickly without added fat. Choose plain boiled rice and cucumber and mint raita, a cooling low-GI accompaniment.
- Avoid the richer dishes such as korma, pasanda, masala, and deep-fried samosas and bhajis. Save your GiPs for bigger portions of better choices.
- Accompany your meal with some steamed or boiled basmati rice, and stay away from pilau and biryanis, unless you only have a small amount.
- Add a GiP-free salad to whatever you're having. In Indian restaurants, they're usually dressed in lime or lemon juice and these acids can help lower the GI of the meal.
- Ask for your popadums to be grilled or

microwaved – they taste just as crunchy as fried ones, and have less than half the fat. You might start a trend, as some restaurants now serve this routinely.

● Now here's a tip. Many Indian restaurants have Bangladeshi owners. Typical Bangladeshi rice has the lowest GI (at least half the GiPs of any other rice). So, ask for it, hype it up, and there'll be more of it on the menu so you can go out for an Indian meal more often!

● Finish with a fresh fruit salad or a standard ice cream. Both are good low-GI options. Indian ice cream (kulfi) is usually made from full-cream milk, cream, sweetened condensed milk and nuts – so leave that for the others.

Remember GiP Rule 5: Have at least one low-GiP food at each meal and always have a snack.

Eating Chinese

A Chinese menu will feature plenty of vegetables, rice and noodles with lots of low-GI, low-fat dishes to choose from. Using chopsticks makes you eat more slowly, so you could end up using fewer GiPs! You might even impress your mates with your new skill …

● Choose healthy starters such as satay dishes with chilli dipping sauces and soups. Avoid deep-fried foods like seaweed and spring rolls.

- Opt for anything on the menu that is steamed, such as whole steamed fish with ginger, steamed vegetables and steamed rice.
- Stir-fried dishes are a great choice, as this method of cooking uses very little oil. Select dishes with added vegetables to keep your GiPs low.
- Jasmine rice is high in GiPs (a whopping 8 points), as is Asian-style sticky rice (7 points). You would be better off with noodles (egg, rice or mung bean – allow 3 GiPs) as a lower-GI alternative. Choose steamed rice rather than special fried varieties.
- For dessert finish with fresh fruit or some canned lychees (leave the syrup).

Eating Thai

Thai dishes can be very healthy. They typically include small amounts of meat, seafood or tofu with vegetables and spicy sauce. Most are good choices. Follow the advice as for Chinese food. Also …

- Avoid the deep-fried starters and go for clear soups, chicken satay or steamed vegetable dumplings, which are lower in fat yet high in taste.
- Thai curries contain coconut cream, which is high in saturated fat. Instead, choose stir-fries or noodle dishes – add some extra chilli sauce if you dare!

EATING OUT THE GiP WAY

Eating French

French restaurants serve many dishes that are generally drenched in rich creamy sauces, but there will always be something on the menu that is healthy or can be made healthier.

● For starters, tuck into a plate of crudités, and choose lower-fat dressings or healthy dips based on tomato or yoghurt. Vegetable soup can be a healthy lower-GI option, but avoid the creamy ones. Remember that the puréed soups will be higher in GI than the more chunky ones. If you're eating bread, select wholegrain bread or a granary roll, or ask for melon or prawn cocktail dressed in lime juice.

● Ask to have your meat or fish grilled without oil, or just a small amount. Avoid the creamy, butter-rich sauces and ask for some fresh lemon wedges or French mustard instead. If you have been given sauce, hide some under that wilted lettuce leaf before you tuck in.

● Choose unbuttered new potatoes with your meal rather than mash, baked potato or French fries. New potatoes have a lower GI. Or go for noodles or couscous instead. Make sure you have heaps of unbuttered vegetables or salad.

● If you're tempted by the dessert menu, make a beeline for sweets with fruit and plain ice cream. Remember, they may still be huge portions, so ask for two spoons and share it with your dinner date.

Eating Mexican

Many of the food choices at Mexican restaurants can be high GI and are often fried or served with creamy sauces, so choose carefully.

- Mexican tortilla wraps score well on the GiP scale. It all depends on what you put in them. Beans are a great low-GiP choice and are filling, so you'll have less room for afters.
- Stick with the grilled seafood and chicken dishes such as fajitas or bean burritos, served with lots of crunchy salad and a fruity tomato or mango salsa. Avoid the sour cream and go easy on the cheese and guacamole. They may have a low GI but they are high in fat, so they aren't GiP-friendly.
- Watch out for the deep-fried taco salad shells – the word 'salad' *doesn't* make it healthy, the word 'fried' *does* mean high fat!
- Avoid the potato wedges: they're laden with calories, particularly when covered in melted cheese and sour cream. Ask for vegetable crudités or a plate of plain corn chips (5 GiPs to share out) with a spicy salsa tomato dip.

Remember GiP Rule 2: Keep as close as you can to your daily GiPs.

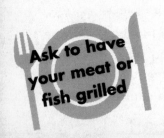

Ask to have your meat or fish grilled

Breakfast at the 'greasy spoon'!

Not the easiest place to find healthier low-GI choices, but here we show you how.

- Rather than a fry-up, try poached egg or baked beans on unbuttered granary toast. Order tomatoes grilled or canned: they're low GI and free of points.
- Some cafés serve porridge or muesli with semi-skimmed milk for breakfast. These are great low-GI cereals to keep your energy levels up throughout the morning.

The party pooper

We've all been there, you get to a party and are faced with a table full of scrummy buffet goodies. It's too tempting to resist and so easy to overindulge! But beware, those tiny nibbles – sausage rolls, vol-au-vents and mini-quiches – are usually loaded with calories and you're less conscious of the calories piling up since they look so small. What do you do?

- Have a low-GiP snack before you get there.
- Reach for the seeded bread or mini pitta sandwiches. Choose those that aren't dripping in mayo. Roast chicken and salad, tuna and sweetcorn or ham and mustard are cool.
- Chicken drumsticks without the skin score well too.

- Having a couple of chipolatas on cocktail sticks isn't the end of the world, but ensure you limit it to a couple.
- If you're lucky, there will be a plate of crunchy salad vegetables and a dip. Have plenty of these but make sure you can still see the carrot when it comes out of the dip! Go for salsa dips and tzatziki.
- Having made your choices, start circulating. You'll be so busy yapping you won't have time to eat!

Eating and drinking

Alcohol is very calorific. An average glass of wine contains more calories than a banana. A measure of spirit has more calories than a packet of Polo mints. A pint of lager has more calories than a small bag of crisps. So, when eating out, watch the amount you drink, as the calories soon clock up. There are loads more GiP tips on alcohol in Chapter 10, but for now try some of these handy hints:

- Drink GiP-free water or a diet soft drink before drinking any alcohol, so that you are not thirsty when you start.

Alcohol: maximum of 7 units for women, 10 units for men per week, in addition to your daily points (see page 192).

- Ask for a jug of water with your meal and drink water between each sip of your alcoholic drink.
- Dilute alcohol, for example by mixing white wine with soda water to make a spritzer, or beer with diet lemonade to make a shandy.
- Make sure you have diet mixers.

On the move with fast food

Fast-food restaurants and cafés can spell trouble for Gippers, but it doesn't mean they're out of bounds.

When a burger calls ...

- A hamburger bun has a higher GI value than seeded bread, so you get 5 GiPs in the bun alone. Add one standard burger and it tots up to 8.5 points. Words like jumbo, giant, deluxe, super-sized mean larger portions, larger GiPs and larger hips. Order a regular hamburger (no cheese) or junior size instead.
- Flavour your burger with sweet and sour, or tomato sauce rather than mayo, and always say 'no' to cheese.
- Veggie doesn't necessarily mean virtuous. Veggie burgers are generally still cooked in fat and served with a creamy sauce.
- Fries clock up 6 on the GiP scale. Thin-cut chips like French fries absorb more fat than thick ones, as there is a larger surface area for the oil to seep into.

A 'regular' portion instead of 'large' could save you half the calories. Ideally, avoid chips if you can.

- Try adding a green salad – avoid the dressing and it's GiP-free. Remember v,v,p,c (page 10).
- Do your belly a favour and choose diet drinks – you can save yourself around 10 teaspoons of sugar by ordering a diet drink instead of a regular one.
- Munch through an apple or banana *before* you visit the burger bar, or order fruit chunks or fresh fruit, if available.

In the sandwich bar

At your local café, pub, sandwich shop, garage or newsagents, sandwiches are readily available and are a quick and easy lunchtime option.

- Opt for bread with seeds or grains.
- Choose lower-GI breads such as wholegrain breads, sourdough, rye bread or granary.
- At a sandwich bar, ask for 'no butter' on your bread.
- Choose lower-fat fillings such as lean meat, chicken or fish with piles of crunchy salad.
- Say 'no' to mayo. Flavour with freshly ground black pepper, mustard, pickles, chutney, salsa or lemon juice.
- Finish off with some fruit and a low-fat yoghurt, two great low-GI desserts.

In the chippy

Let's face it, if you're in the chippy you are there to buy chips! Chips are high GI and high fat, so not ideal. Is there a healthier solution?

- Order a small portion and be careful what you choose to eat them with. Or make a chip butty with granary bread (and no butter!).
- Leave the batter – just eat the fish inside.
- Rather than sausages or meat pasties, choose a piece of chicken (remove the skin), and have some mushy peas, if available. (Mushy peas are higher in GI than whole peas, but some peas are better than none.)
- How about filling up on a pickled egg or pickled onions and having fewer chips?
- Some outlets offer shish kebabs and salad, which are healthier options.

In the kebab joint

Kebabs can be healthy and filling, provided the meat is lean. Pitta bread generally has a lower GI than some other breads, so you get more for your GiPs (one whole pitta has half a point less than a couple of slices of white bread and is more filling).

Go for tandoori chicken, chicken tikka, char-grilled kebabs and piles of salad

- Avoid doner kebab – have you seen the fat drip down and congeal at the bottom? Shish kebab is better because the chunks of meat are leaner to start with and are then char-grilled, which allows the fat to drain off. You can also get minced beef kebabs and, again, since they are char-grilled, you do lose some of the fat. Have pitta bread, stuffed with salad.
- A veggie option, such as falafel, is usually deep-fried, so they're not necessarily lower in calories. Have fewer falafel or a small amount of hummus and fill the pitta bread with tzatziki and loads of salad.
- Another choice is to go for the char-grilled vegetable kebab. Ask for peppers and other veggies to be threaded on to skewers, flavoured with their sauces and then char-grilled. Pile this into pitta bread along with salad, and indulge – safe in the knowledge that you've gone for the healthy option.

Spuds

Jacket potatoes have a high GI but you can lower the GI of the overall meal by choosing lower-GI fillings:

- Ask for no butter.
- Good fillings include baked beans (with a small sprinkling of grated cheese if you need it); chilli con carne with kidney beans; tuna and sweetcorn (no mayo); coleslaw and beans; cottage cheese and salad. See the Lunch Combos for points value of some baked potato meals (pages 85 and 307).

When you become crystal clear about adopting and adapting to a healthy lifestyle, you increase the likelihood of succeeding.

Once in a while you will have to choose foods that are not so healthy. When this happens, remember that one unhealthy meal is not a disaster. You are not going to pile on the pounds by eating this one meal. You can always compensate by making sure your other meals that day, or the day after, contain healthier low-GiP foods. Remember, eating out is all part of the fun GiP lifestyle.

Are you a Real Gipper?

Question:

Are you conscious of the types of fat you eat?

Choice 1: I eat fatty meats and full-fat dairy products because I can't resist them.

It's fine to choose these foods, just watch how often. If you overdo such high-animal-fat foods, you are more likely to gain weight and risk raised blood cholesterol.

Choice 2: I choose foods and cooking methods that are low in fat.

As part of an overall healthy lifestyle, these foods

help you keep in shape and support your Gi Point Diet and general health.

Choice 3: I eat oily fish once a week.

The special omega-3 fats in oily fish protect against heart disease and are in keeping with your GiPs. Consequently, choosing oily fish on a weekly basis simply reduces your risks.

Results:

Choice 1: Eating as you've always done can only lead to the same results. If you don't like what you're experiencing, change it NOW!

Choice 2: Making well-informed choices today will shape your life tomorrow. Life is a building process – each small action has an accumulative effect.

Choice 3: Celebrate your choice here and keep reminding yourself of the rewards that this brings!

So be a Real Gipper – and choose in line with the new you.

Summary

- Eating out is one of the continued pleasures of life on the GiP plan.
- Your choices today will shape your life tomorrow.
- Choose lower-GI breads with lower-fat fillings.

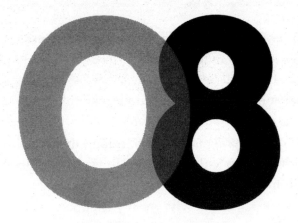

TASTY
GiP RECIPES

Starters or side dishes

Baked Tiger Prawns
(1 point per serving)

You can use any type of prawn or seafood for this dish, but tiger prawns add that special touch.

Serves 4

15 ml/1 tbsp olive oil

2 cloves garlic, peeled and sliced thinly

225 g/8 oz large raw prawns (such as tiger prawns),
peeled and heads removed

Garnish:

Freshly chopped parsley

½ lemon, cut into wedges

1 Preheat the oven to 200°C/400°F/Gas Mark 6.

2 Put the olive oil and garlic in a large, shallow, oven-proof dish and heat in the oven for 2–3 minutes until very hot. You need to watch this carefully so that the garlic does not start to brown.

3 Add the prawns carefully, rolling them in the hot oil, and return to the oven for a further 3 minutes until they are pink and cooked.

4 Serve, sprinkled with freshly chopped parsley and lemon wedges for squeezing.

Chilli and Honey Chicken Wings
(2 points per serving)

Although this is basted with olive oil, the chicken wings are skinless, so this helps to cut down on saturated fat. Finger-lickin' good, just remember to serve this with plenty of napkins!

Serves 4

12 skinless chicken wings
2.5 cm/1 in stick root ginger, crushed
2 cloves garlic, crushed
5 ml/1 tsp red chilli powder
15 ml/1 tbsp olive oil
10 ml/2 tsp runny honey
10 ml/2 tsp coarse-grain mustard
5 ml/1 tsp cider vinegar
Salt and pepper

1 Preheat the grill to medium. Line a large flame-proof dish with foil.

2 Put the wings into a bowl. Add all the other ingredients and mix well.

3 Arrange the chicken wings in the dish, making sure they don't overlap.

4 Cook under the grill for about 20 minutes, turning once or twice during cooking. Serve hot or cold.

Beef Tomatoes with Black Olives
(1 point per serving)

Serves 4

8 beef tomatoes, sliced
12 pitted black olives, halved
Paprika and garlic salt, to taste
15 ml/1 tbsp olive oil
2 spring onions, sliced

1 Preheat the oven to 200°C/400°F/Gas 6. Lightly grease an ovenproof dish.

2 Layer the tomatoes with the olives in the dish and season with the paprika and garlic salt.

3 Drizzle on the olive oil and place in the middle shelf of the oven until soft but not mushy. Garnish with the spring onions and serve warm.

Char-grilled Vegetables with Honey and Basil *(2 points per serving)*

Serves 4
10 ml/2 tsp rapeseed oil
2 courgettes, sliced
1 green pepper, sliced
1 aubergine, sliced
2 tomatoes, halved and sliced
30 ml/2 tbsp balsamic vinegar
5 ml/1 tsp honey
Handful of fresh basil leaves, torn, or ½ tsp dried basil
Sprinkling of salt and ground black pepper

1 Preheat the grill. Line a baking tray or grill pan with foil and drizzle one teaspoon of oil over it.
2 Place all the vegetables in a single layer over the oil.
3 Cover the vegetables with the remaining ingredients and grill under a medium heat for 15 minutes, turning frequently till the vegetables are softened and browned. Serve immediately.

Curried Cauliflower
(1 point per serving)

A simple way to spice up vegetables such as cauliflower, broccoli or cabbage. You can add some chilli sauce for extra zing.

Serves 4

30 ml/2 tbsp rapeseed oil
10 ml/2 tsp black mustard seeds
5 ml/1 tsp cumin seeds
1 cauliflower, cut into florets
1 tsp curry powder
Good pinch of red chilli powder
15 ml/1 tbsp mixed freshly chopped herbs
60 ml/4 tbsp water
Salt and pepper to taste

1 Heat the oil in a wok or a frying pan with a lid.

2 Add the mustard and cumin seeds until they start to pop. This will only take a few seconds.

3 Add the cauliflower and cook, stirring, for about 5 minutes.

4 Add the remaining ingredients, cover and cook for 10 minutes or until the cauliflower is tender but still crunchy.

Layered Mushroom and Tomato with Grilled Cheese (1 point per serving)

A starter or side dish that goes with most meals. Just wait for the aroma and the sight of melting cheese dripping down the vegetables and tingling those taste buds. This dish also works well with a range of vegetables.

Serves 4

4 large mushrooms
Pinch dried mixed herbs
Salt and black pepper
1 large tomato, cut into 4 slices
50 g/1½ oz half-fat Cheddar cheese, grated
Mustard and cress

1 Preheat the oven to 190°C/375°F/Gas Mark 5.

2 Put the mushrooms flat side up on a non-stick baking tray.

3 Sprinkle some mixed herbs and seasoning over the mushrooms and top with a tomato slice.

4 Bake in the oven for 25 minutes. Preheat the grill.

5 Sprinkle grated cheese over each mushroom and place under a hot grill until the cheese has melted.

6 Sprinkle over the mustard and cress and serve.

Middle Eastern Tabouleh Salad
(3 points per serving)

A Lebanese herby salad that goes well with kebabs and tzatziki (Greek yoghurt with cucumber, garlic and mint) or indeed with simple grilled fish.

Serves 4

100 g/3½ oz bulgur wheat, pre-soaked in hot water for 1 hour, drained
100 g/3½ oz flat-leaf parsley, chopped roughly
5 tomatoes, diced
25 g/1 oz mint leaves (chopped)
25 g/1 oz coriander leaves (chopped)
1 onion, finely chopped
For the dressing:
Pinch of salt
Pinch of ground allspice
Pinch of ground cinnamon
Juice of 2 lemons
30 ml/2 tbsp olive oil

1 First make the dressing. Put all the dressing ingredients in a screw-top jar, cover and shake vigorously.
2 Mix the soaked wheat with the parsley, tomatoes, mint, coriander and onion.
3 Toss in the dressing and serve.

Kidney Bean and Chick Pea Salad in Mustard Dressing (2.5 points per serving)

An unusual accompaniment to meat or fish – no need to add extra carbs as there are already some in the beans.

Serves 4

2 green peppers
30 g/1 oz of fresh chives, snipped
6 spring onions, roots removed and chopped finely
200 g/7 oz can red kidney beans, drained
400 g/14 oz can chick peas, drained
1 red onion, chopped

Dressing:

20 ml/1½ tbsp olive oil
Juice of 1 small lemon
1 clove garlic, peeled and crushed
10 ml/2 tsp wholegrain French mustard
½ tsp mixed dried herbs

1 Spear the peppers with a fork and hold over a gas flame (or under a hot grill) until the skins are blackened all over.

2 Remove the skins and the seeds, then dice and place in a large bowl.

3 Add the chives, spring onions, kidney beans, chickpeas and red onion, and mix well.

4 Make the dressing. Put all the dressing ingredients in a screw-top jar, cover and shake vigorously.

5 Pour this over the salad and mix well.

6 Cover with cling film and chill for at least 15 minutes before serving.

Chilli Peanut Popcorn
(2.5 points)

A crunchy snack for those *curled-up-on-the-sofa* video nights. Remember that this counts as your once-a-day nut allowance, so be sure not to have peanut butter or any other nuts on the same day.

Serves 3

50 g/2 oz salted peanuts
½ tsp red chilli powder
½ tsp corn oil
2 tbsp (25 g) popping corn
Lemon juice, to taste

1 Heat a heavy-based pan with a lid, add the peanuts and toss them over a medium heat until lightly toasted.

2 Remove from the heat and place the peanuts in a bowl. While still warm, sprinkle over the red chilli powder and stir well.

3 Pour the oil into the pan and, when heated, add the popping corn and cover. Maintain on a medium heat. The corn should start to pop and hit the lid.

4 Remove from heat once the popping stops and pour the popped corn into the bowl with the peanuts. Stir well, add more chilli powder if desired and lemon juice to taste just before serving.

(Recipe courtesy of the National Peanut Board.)

Main meals

Cod Kebabs with Fresh Dill
(1.5 points per serving)

Serves 4
650 g/1 lb 7 oz cod fillet
15 ml/1 tbsp olive oil
2 cloves garlic, crushed
Zest and juice of 1 lemon
30 ml/2 tbsp freshly chopped dill
30 ml/2 tbsp freshly chopped coriander leaves
Salt and black pepper
2 limes, quartered
Cherry tomatoes, to serve

1 Cut the fish into chunks and place in a bowl with the olive oil, garlic, lemon zest and juice, dill, coriander and seasoning. Stir well.
2 Pre-heat the grill to medium and line a grill pan with foil.
3 Thread the fish pieces on to four skewers and secure the ends with the lime wedges.
4 Grill, turning occasionally, for about 5–8 minutes. Serve with halved cherry tomatoes.

Salmon Steaks in Garlicky Balsamic Vinegar
(3.5 points per serving)

You can prepare this dish in the same amount of time as it takes to lay the table – literally 5 minutes! The salmon is smothered in a mixture of fresh garlic, soy sauce, coarse-grain mustard and balsamic vinegar, and grilled quickly. (Alternatively, try wrapping the fish in foil with a sprig of fresh dill and some chopped spring onions, and cook in a moderate oven.) Serve on a bed of brown rice, with a crisp green salad, and for that really special occasion, partner it with asparagus tips.

Serves 4

4 salmon steaks, each about 175 g/6 oz
30 ml/2 tbsp balsamic vinegar
30 ml/2 tbsp soy sauce
15 ml/1 tbsp olive oil
2 heaped tsp coarse-grain mustard
2 garlic cloves, crushed
30 ml/2 tbsp fresh dill, finely chopped
Salt and freshly milled black pepper

1 Place the salmon steaks in a non-metallic dish. Mix together the vinegar, soy sauce, olive oil, mustard, garlic, dill and seasoning.

2 Pour the sauce over the salmon, turning to coat. If marinating, cover and leave in the refrigerator for 30 minutes.

3 Preheat the grill. Lift the salmon out of the marinade and place on a foil-lined grill pan. Coat the steaks with the sauce and grill under a moderate heat for 4–5 minutes each side.

Haddock with Thai Green Pepper and Basil Sauce (2.5 points per serving)

You can use any white fish for this dish, though haddock or cod fillets work especially well. The green pepper and basil are combined with a Thai green curry paste to make an unusual and exciting blend of flavours.

Serves 4

4 haddock fillets, about 175 g/6 oz each
15 ml/1 tbsp olive oil
5 ml/1 tsp crushed garlic
5 ml/1 tsp crushed ginger
Salt and coarse black pepper

For the sauce:

3 green peppers, halved and deseeded
10 ml/2 tsp olive oil
1 onion, chopped
10 ml/2 tsp Thai green curry paste
Few fresh basil leaves, torn
1 sprig of fresh thyme or a pinch of dried thyme
30 ml/2 tbsp lime juice

To garnish:

Few sprigs of fresh coriander

1 Preheat the grill. Place the peppers, skin side up, on a baking sheet. Cook under a hot grill until the skins are blackened. Leave aside to cool.

2 Brush the fish lightly on both sides with the olive oil, and spread with garlic and ginger. Season and place on a foiled grill pan. Grill, turning once, until the fish flakes easily (about 10–12 minutes).

3 Now make the sauce. Heat the oil and sauté the chopped onions until translucent, about 2–3 minutes. Add the curry paste and cook for a further minute.

4 Peel the peppers and place them in a food processor with the onion mixture, herbs and lime juice. Blend until smooth. Adjust the seasoning if necessary.

5 Serve the fish with the green pepper sauce, garnished with fresh coriander.

Instant Noodles with Prawns and Garlic
(6.5 points per serving)

Simply boil the noodles, stir-fry some prawns, and there you have it: a Chinese meal good enough to take away!

Serves 4

350 g/12½ oz instant noodles
30 ml/2 tbsp vegetable oil
200 g/7 oz frozen prawns, thawed and drained
2 cloves garlic, finely chopped
45 ml/3 tbsp sun-dried tomato paste
200 g/7 oz cherry tomatoes
Salt and freshly ground pepper

1 Cook the noodles in a large saucepan of boiling water, following the instructions on the packet.

2 Heat the oil in a large frying pan. Add the prawns and the garlic. Stir-fry on medium heat for 3–5 minutes.

3 Stir in the tomato paste and mix well. To this add 30 ml/2 tbsp of water. Add the cherry tomatoes and stir gently.

4 Toss this into the drained noodles. Season to taste.

Sweet and Sour Chicken Drumsticks
(3 points per serving)

These sticky drumsticks are delicious with Hot Roasted Vegetables (free snack – page 149) and sweet potatoes.

Serves 4

4 chicken drumsticks, skinned
30 ml/2 tbsp runny honey
15 ml/1 tbsp sesame oil
45 ml/3 tbsp low-sodium soy sauce
30 ml/2 tbsp lemon juice
10 ml/2 tsp coarse-grain mustard

1 Preheat the oven to 200°C/400°F/Gas Mark 6. Pierce the drumsticks with a skewer or fork to allow the flavours to penetrate.

2 Mix together the honey, sesame oil, soy sauce, lemon juice and mustard. Place the chicken into a lightly greased oven-proof dish and spread this mixture evenly over the chicken.

3 Cook for 25–30 minutes till the juices run clear when you pierce the chicken with a fork. Serve hot or cold.

Sizzling Turkey Burgers
(1.5 points per serving)

On days when there's only boring ordinary mince in the fridge, these hot and spicy burgers will make your mouth water. Speedy turkey burgers make a change from beef or chicken burgers, and all you have to do is mix all the ingredients together and grill! Great with salads, and if you're serving them with hamburger buns add 5 points per bun.

Serves 4 (makes 8 burgers)

450 g/1 lb minced turkey
1 onion, grated
2 cloves garlic, crushed
5 ml/1 tsp paprika
Salt and pepper

1 Preheat the grill to medium.
2 Mix all the ingredients together.
3 Shape the mixture into 8 burgers.
4 Grill under medium heat for 4–5 minutes each side until the meat is cooked.

Turkey Stroganoff
(1.5 points per serving)

A lower-fat version of the traditional stroganoff. Serve with basmati rice (remember to add the points) and a fresh herb salad.

Serves 4

Spray oil
500 g/1 lb 2 oz turkey breast, diced into chunks
2 small onions, thinly sliced
30 ml/2 tbsp mint sauce
100 ml/4 tbsp low-fat natural yoghurt
Salt and pepper
Fresh coriander leaves, to garnish

1 Heat 5 sprays of oil in a non-stick pan and fry the turkey pieces until lightly coloured.

2 Add the onions and stir the mixture until lightly browned.

3 Stir in the remaining ingredients and gently bring to the boil, stirring all the time to prevent curdling.

4 Cover and simmer on low heat until the meat is cooked. Season and garnish with coriander.

Cheesy Pork Chops
(2.5 points per serving)

An unusual combination, grilled or pan-fried pork chops are topped with a mustard cheese sauce. Serve with lightly cooked green vegetables and potatoes of your choice.

Serves 2

1 clove garlic, crushed
A little salt
½ tsp black peppercorns, coarsely ground
½ tsp dried rosemary
½ tsp dried thyme
Juice of 1 lemon
2 pork chops, fat removed
25 g/1 oz reduced-fat Cheddar cheese, grated
½ tsp English mustard

1 Mix the garlic, salt, pepper, rosemary and lemon juice. Rub this over both sides of the pork chops. Leave covered in the fridge for 1 hour.

2 Heat the griddle pan to very hot and grill each chop for 7 minutes on each side.

3 Mix the cheese with the mustard. Spread this over the chops. Grill the chops until the cheese is golden brown.

Herby Pork Chops
(2 points per serving)

You can use any herbs you like for this dish, but this combination is especially tasty. Partner these herby chops with some Savoy Cabbage with Caraway Seeds (free snack – page 148) and lightly cooked fettuccine (1.5 points extra).

Serves 4

4 pork chops, lean
Salt and coarsely ground black pepper
5 ml/1 tsp dried oregano
5 ml/1 tsp dried marjoram
Juice of 1 lemon
Spray oil

1 Preheat the grill.
2 Sprinkle both sides of the chops with all the ingredients and spray with oil (about 2 sprays each side per chop).
3 Place under the grill in medium heat for 7–8 minutes each side or until meat is cooked.

Beef Chow Mein
(7 points per serving)

This tangy dish is delicious for a special occasion or for an evening meal where you have those insatiable hunger pangs. The beef is cut into thin strips so it takes very little time to cook. Noodles and other pasta have a low Glycaemic Index. Serve with masses of vegetables.

Serves 4

45 ml/3 tbsp soy sauce

450 g/16 oz rump steak, cut into thin strips

2.5 cm/1 in piece root ginger, peeled and sliced
into thin strips

350 g/12 oz instant noodles

30 ml/2 tbsp rapeseed oil

1 onion, thinly sliced

1 green or red pepper, cut into chunks

75 g/2½ oz button mushrooms

2 large tomatoes, cut into wedges

10 ml/2 tsp rapeseed oil

Salt and pepper

1 Drizzle the soy sauce over the beef, add the ginger and, if you have time, leave to marinate for 30 minutes. Drain the beef, reserving the marinade.

2 Cook the noodles in a large saucepan of boiling water, following the instructions on the packet. Drain and set aside.

3 Heat 30 ml/2 tbsp oil in a wok and stir-fry the meat for 2−3 minutes on high. Remove with a slotted spoon and keep warm.

4 Add the onion, pepper and mushrooms and stir-fry for 4 minutes. Next add the marinade, cooked beef and the tomato wedges. Cook for 2–3 minutes until the vegetables are cooked but crisp.

5 Heat 10 ml/2 tsp of rapeseed oil in a wok or large pan. Stir in the noodles, season and serve with the beef.

Couscous with Peppers and Red Onion
(4.5 points per serving)

Couscous makes a refreshing change from potatoes, rice and pasta. In this recipe, it is mixed with crunchy chopped peppers, flat-leaf parsley and red onion to give a flavoursome carb accompaniment to any meal. It can be served hot or cold (as in this recipe) and can be bought in flavoured varieties, such as lemon and garlic. This recipe can be made up to 24 hours in advance and kept covered in the fridge until needed.

Serves 4 as main course, 6–8 as an accompaniment
(18 points for total recipe)

225 g/8 oz couscous
20 ml/4 tsp olive oil
Juice of 1 lime
3 small mixed peppers, de-seeded and finely chopped
1 small red onion, finely chopped
Bunch of flat-leaf parsley (about 80 g/3 oz), washed and roughly chopped (remove any tough stalks as necessary)

1 Put the dry couscous in a large mixing bowl.
2 Add the same amount of boiling water (225 ml/ 8 fl oz) and stir briefly with a fork.
3 Stir in the olive oil and lime juice.
4 Add the chopped peppers, onion and flat-leaf parsley leaves and mix well.
5 Leave, out of the fridge, for 30 minutes for the flavours to develop and mingle.

Mediterranean Pasta
(5 points per serving)

The smell of fresh garlic … the crunch of lightly cooked vegetables … the colours of the Mediterranean. This delicious Italian meal is a filling family favourite, which goes well with a simple green salad.

Serves 4

45 ml/3 tbsp olive oil
2 mixed (or 1 green, 1 red) peppers, diced
3 courgettes, sliced thinly, diagonally
1½ tsp dried oregano
2 bay leaves
3 tomatoes, cut into eighths
240 g/8½ oz dried pasta (penne, for example)
3 cloves garlic, crushed
1 onion, finely chopped
450 g/1 lb mushrooms, sliced
Salt and coarsely ground black pepper
15 ml/1 tbsp fresh parsley, finely chopped

1 Preheat the oven to 240°C/475°F/Gas Mark 9. Drizzle a teaspoon of oil into a large roasting tin. Layer the peppers and courgettes into the pan, adding the oregano, bay leaves and seasoning in between the layers. Drizzle the remaining oil over the vegetables, saving about two teaspoons of oil for the pasta.

2 Bake uncovered at the top of the oven for 20–25 minutes, until slightly charred, adding the tomatoes after about 15 minutes. Stir once during cooking.

3 Cook the pasta in lightly salted water according to the instructions on the packet (around 10 minutes).

4 Meanwhile, heat the remaining oil in a large non-stick pan. Add the garlic, onion and mushrooms and fry until the onions are light brown and the mushrooms are just cooked.

5 Take the vegetables out of the oven, stir gently and mix thoroughly with the pasta and the mushrooms and onion mixture. Adjust the seasoning if necessary, and sprinkle with parsley.

Speedy GiP-free snacks

Garlic Mushrooms

Put some button mushrooms into a pan with low-sodium soy sauce, garlic purée, cracked black pepper and any dried herbs you have lying around. Throw in chopped spring onions or chives. Cook quickly and eat slowly.

Cabbage with Fennel Seeds

Steam some cabbage, or raid the fridge for leftover GiP-free vegetables. Warm a frying pan and pour in a little balsamic vinegar. Add the cabbage, a teaspoon of fennel seeds, a pinch of cayenne pepper, a touch of salt and some ground black pepper.

Grilled Tomato Salad

Slice a large tomato, season with paprika and garlic salt. Place under a preheated grill till charred, top with chopped red onion.

Courgette Boats

Halve a courgette lengthways. Flavour with black pepper, ground cumin or curry powder. Add a little salt and some lemon juice. Microwave until just cooked – about a minute or so.

Chilli and Lime Rocket Leaves

Mix together your favourite combination of GiP-free salad veggies and rocket leaves. Make a dressing using fresh lime juice, paprika, dried herbs and chilli sauce. Drench and devour.

Warming Marrow and Leek Soup

Throw together some chopped marrow, diced red peppers and leeks. Heat a pan with 300 ml (½ pint) of water, made up to stock using half a stock cube (or less). Add the vegetables with a large pinch of dried parsley, cook through and add pepper to taste.

Savoy Cabbage with Caraway Seeds

Steam about 150 g/5 oz cabbage quickly until just cooked. Drain. Add five sprays of spray oil to a non-stick frying pan. Heat the oil and add the cabbage. Stir-fry over a high heat with a teaspoon of caraway seeds, season, sprinkle on some cayenne pepper and serve.

Herby Baby Spinach and Beansprouts

Simply mix the spinach and beansprouts together and flavour with fresh flat-leaf parsley, rice vinegar and paprika.

Gherkin and Onion Pickle

Chop some gherkins; add a halved pickled onion or two, sprinkle on some red chilli powder.

Stir-fried Babycorn

Heat a pan with five sprays of oil. Chuck in some baby sweetcorn, season with a little soy sauce and black pepper.

Curried Okra

Heat five sprays of spray oil and add a good pinch of cumin seeds. Let them pop for a few seconds over a low heat to release the aroma. Add a couple of teaspoons of tomato purée and a good pinch of curry powder. Blend together over a low heat – add some water if it sticks to the bottom. Pile in some boiled or canned okra and some diced red onion or spring onions. Smother in freshly chopped coriander.

Balsamic French Beans

Boil the French beans until just cooked. Drain and add balsamic vinegar and a little salt to taste.

Hot Roasted Vegetables

Mix together your favourite combination of chopped peppers, mushrooms, onions, courgettes, asparagus, celery, baby corn and tomatoes. Add a teaspoon or so of crushed garlic, some fresh or dried herbs, a little salt and pepper. Place in a foil-lined tray and bake in a hot oven till cooked (about 15 minutes).

Speedy Salsa Sauce

Heat five sprays of spray oil in a non-stick frying pan and add a crushed clove of garlic. Stir-fry some finely chopped onion and green or red pepper. Add a couple of chopped canned tomatoes with some of the tomato juice and flavour with a good pinch of red chilli powder. Simmer for about 5 minutes.

Cucumber and Mint Cooler
Cut some chilled cucumber into wedges and top with chopped fresh mint, lemon juice and coarsely ground black pepper.

Spiced Vegetables
Choose your favourite GiP-free raw or cooked vegetables and add a good pinch each of curry powder, paprika and ground cumin with a touch of salt.

Al Dente Asparagus
Steam asparagus tips with a little crushed garlic till lightly cooked. Season lightly and serve immediately.

Wheat-free Tabouleh
First make the dressing. Put a pinch each of salt, ground allspice and ground cinnamon and some lemon juice into a screw-top jar, cover and shake vigorously. Mix together roughly chopped flat-leaf parsley, diced tomatoes, chopped mint leaves and a finely chopped onion. Toss in the dressing and serve.

Jelly with Whole Strawberries
Make up a sugar-free jelly and add a cupful of fresh strawberries, before the jelly sets completely. Leave to set and chill in the fridge. Alternatively, buy an individual pot of sugar-free jelly, cut it into rough chunks and serve with fresh strawberries.

PART TWO

A HEALTHY BODY AND MIND

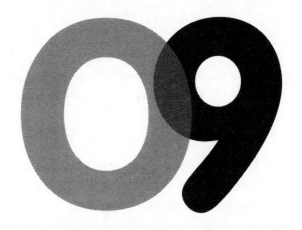

EATING FOR COMPLETE HEALTH

The balance of good health

The GiP plan is your new way of life and, for it to be balanced and sustainable, it is crucial to include foods that provide the range of nutrients that enhance your overall sense of vitality and well-being. And since feeling great isn't only about what's on your plate, this chapter helps you incorporate other aspects of feeling good that are practical enough for the whole family.

Read on for a simple guide to which foods are good for you and why. You'll find lots of healthy eating tips, so just pick out the changes that you feel will easily fit

> There's no need to think that there are foods you must eat and those you must not. Healthy eating is all about balance – choosing a variety of healthy foods you enjoy and not forcing yourself to eat foods you dislike.

into your lifestyle. Indeed, you may find that you are already choosing many of the recommended foods, so eating well may be easier than you think.

Open up any magazine and you'll read about the latest trendy diet, food fads and food scares. The messages are frequently conflicting or misleading – how do you know what is based on good science?

That's where the UK's national food guide, *The Balance of Good Health*, comes in. Eating well is like a buffet – pick 'n' choose what you like, but be aware of its effect on you, be it emotionally (a pat on the back) or physically (a leaner and fitter you).

The Balance of Good Health, produced by the Food Standards Agency, is a simple and practical tool to help you eat a range of foods in the optimum amounts. The guide is made up of five food groups, each group representing a different segment on the plate. Notice that these vary in size, depending on the proportions needed to make up a healthy diet.

What are the five food groups?

● Bread, cereals (such as breakfast cereals) and starchy foods (such as potatoes, pasta and rice).

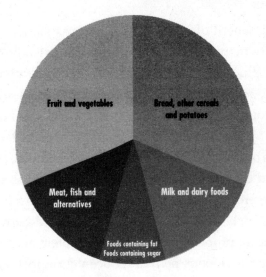

- Fruit and vegetables.
- Dairy products, such as milk and cheese.
- Meat, fish and alternatives, such as soya, beans and nuts.
- Fatty and sugary foods.

Remember GiP Rule 8: Choose a balanced day by having a variety of foods from the different food groups.

Bread, cereals and starchy foods

Love your carbs? No problem. You can devour them on this diet – from fruit loaf to fettuccine, since low-GiP carbs are all part of that buffet.

Starchy foods, such as bread, rice, potatoes and pasta, are great energy providers. GiP eating has the added benefit of pointing you to those starchy foods that are more likely to give you a slow, steady rise in blood glucose. These 'right carbs' not only give you energy but also fill you up. That's because these foods take longer to digest, so you don't feel the need to reach for that extra helping or raid the fridge later.

Carbs also provide a wide range of vitamins, minerals and dietary fibre. Carbs can even be a good source of protein. You don't usually think of bread as a protein-rich food, but two slices of bread provide a significant proportion of your daily protein needs. And since protein foods help to reduce your appetite, low-GiP protein foods, like beans, make even more sense.

At one time, carbs may have been thought of as the villains, as many people assumed these foods were fattening. In fact it's not the starchy foods that make you put on weight but the fatty toppings, dressings and sauces you serve with them. So, grainy bread is a great choice, but smother it in butter and it ends up on your hips or belly.

Some recipes in this book contain noodles or pasta, which are excellent starchy foods for Gippers. Pasta is slowly absorbed by the body, so that it will not raise your blood-glucose levels too quickly. If you keep an eye on added fat in cooking, this will mean even more success on your bathroom scales. When you've exhausted the range of things you can do with pasta and noodles there's still basmati rice, couscous, bulgur wheat, oats, sweet potatoes, yams, chapattis, tortillas and much more to get your teeth into.

You can have virtually any carbs you like so long as you pay attention to the GiPs. For example, if you're a potato addict, you'd do well to choose boiled new potatoes in their skins (3 points) rather than a jacket (7 points). Similarly, basmati rice would come top of your shopping list when you fancy a curry or Chinese meal. If you can get hold of Bangladeshi rice (1.5 points) that's even better. Here are some more GiP tips:

Hints and tips

- Serve some low-GiP carbs at every meal. Remember that adding butter or margarine uses up more GiPs.
- Pile your bread bin with low-GiP choices such as tortilla wraps, seeded breads (like multigrain or sunflower seed bread) and fruit loaf.
- Experiment with a wider range of starchy vegetables such as cassava, yams, sweet potatoes and plantains.
- Try basmati rice and couscous for a change.
- Most types of pasta are low in GiPs – make these your regular buddies. Keep the sauce simple. Tomatoes, onions, garlic and peppers don't need much more than a sprinkling of Parmesan cheese and freshly ground black pepper.
- Think 'right carbs'.

The fibre fill-up

Wholegrain varieties of bread and cereals as well as the skin on potatoes are high in fibre. High-fibre starchy foods, such as bran-based cereals and stone-ground wholemeal bread, also help prevent constipation. A simple way of checking if you're eating enough fibre is to check your stools! If they float in the loo bowl you're okay; if not, try a bowl of wholegrain breakfast cereal a day and more fruit and vegetables, drink loads of water, and watch 'em float over the next few days.

It's important to drink plenty of water to help the fibre do its job. Try to have at least six to eight glasses of fluid (such as water or low-calorie drinks) each day.

Oat-based cereals such as porridge and muesli are high in a particular type of fibre called soluble fibre. These foods are even more slowly absorbed than starchy foods in general, which means they are ideal in GiP-eating. What's more, research shows that they can help reduce blood cholesterol. Try to use oats in recipes or start the day with an oat-based cereal. Instant hot oat cereals do contain soluble fibre, but because the oats have been mashed up, they raise blood glucose more rapidly than other types. Go for oats with large flakes instead.

Remember GiP Rule 1: Eat three meals and three snacks every day.

Spread your intake of starchy foods evenly throughout the day and eat regular meals and snacks.

This helps to reduce fluctuations in your blood-glucose levels.

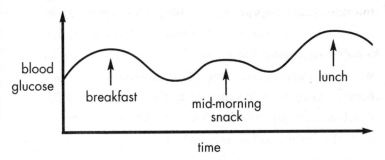

Fruit and vegetables

What do you do if your get-up-and-go just got up and went? Well, the answer is 'Give me five' – fruit and vegetables, that is. In fact, this advice makes so much sense that you'll not only experience a boost of vitality, the extra vitamins and minerals you take in will help build a sound nutritional barrier against cancer and other diseases. And the best news is that most fruit and veg are low in points. Weight loss never tasted so good!

How much is enough?

For good health, you should aim for five 80 g (3 oz) portions a day. Potatoes are classified as starchy carbohydrates, so they don't count. To help people put this into practice, The British Dietetic Association ran a three-year *Food First Campaign* called 'Give Me Five'. Research shows that although people know that fruit and vegetables are healthy, they are less aware of how much of them to eat or the specific benefits they provide.

What's in a portion?
- Medium apple, pear, orange or banana
- Large slice of melon or pineapple
- A teacupful of strawberries or grapes
- ½–1 tablespoon of dried fruit
- 1 small glass of fresh fruit juice
- 2–3 tablespoons of cooked vegetables
- A small serving of salad vegetables, such as a carrot, a tomato or a small bowl of mixed salad
- 2–3 tablespoons of canned vegetables, such as sweetcorn or baked beans

What about juice, dried fruit and veggies in ready meals?
As you can see from the list, dried fruit and fresh fruit juice do count. However, it is best to choose juice as only one of your five portions, since the valuable fibre has been removed. And since juice generally makes your blood glucose rise more quickly than the whole fruit, it's best to have it with a meal so that the rise is evened out by other foods eaten at the same time. Pulses (such as beans and lentils) are also counted just once a day. This is because they don't contain the range of nutrients you get from other foods such as green leafy vegetables, carrots and tomatoes.

So, about half a can of baked beans counts as a portion, and interestingly, since there might well be 80 g (3 oz) of tomatoes in a portion of tomato-based pasta sauce or 80 g of vegetables in a bought stir-fry, then you can, in theory, achieve your five-a-day target by eating bought foods. However, it makes good nutritional sense to have a mixture, to be sure of getting all the nutrients you need, especially since processed foods may be high in salt. Check out the Smart Shopping chapter (page 55) for some low-GiP fruit and veggies.

If you're not keen on cabbage and broccoli don't despair. It's all about variety and choosing foods you enjoy. For example, try using a thin pizza base and smothering it in spinach, peppers, tomatoes, onions and garlic. Fruit smoothies made with liquidised fruit and semi-skimmed milk are another great way to get an extra couple of portions of fruit in.

'Antioxidants' – that magic word

These are natural substances found in fruit, vegetables and some nuts. They include vital vitamins such as vitamins A, C and E as well as lycopene (concentrated in tomatoes), flavenoids (found in tea) and the mineral selenium (found especially in Brazil nuts).

Antioxidants are thought to be protective since they 'mop up' the free radicals, which lurk around in the body and have been linked to premature ageing, heart disease and cancer. Free radicals are produced by normal body processes, but cigarette smoke, ultra-violet light, illness and pollution appear to increase their production. Vitamins have many other health-giving properties. For example, vitamin E can help to strengthen the blood vessels. Vitamin C helps you to absorb iron, which is needed for healthy red blood cells and to prevent anaemia, so have a couple of satsumas or other citrus fruit after a meal that contains iron-rich foods such as meat or broccoli.

And the antioxidant lycopene, concentrated in tomatoes, becomes more potent when the tomatoes are processed. So smothering pasta with a jar of tomato-based pasta sauce might be cheating in the kitchen, but be smug that your meal is packed with hidden bene-fits. And mixing a chunky sauce with low-GI boiled pasta helps you to keep the GI low.

Rainbow eating

The brightly coloured red, yellow and orange veggies are particularly rich in antioxidants, especially beta-carotene. Packed with cancer-fighting power, these 'phytochemicals' are present in fresh fruit and vegeta-bles in precisely the quantities and combination Mother Nature intended. So, taking a supplement containing one or two of them just won't do the trick, compared with the combination found in the real foods. Get into the habit of surveying the natural colours on your plate – the more varied the colours, the more varied the nutrients. Easy as pie! Generally

Dark green fruit and vegetables

Vitamin A   Cabbage, broccoli, spinach, lettuce, parsley and green peppers

Vitamin B   Cabbage, broccoli, spinach, spring greens, green peppers, watercress and parsley

Vitamin E   Broccoli, spinach, spring greens, green peppers, watercress and parsley

Vitamin K   Most green leafy vegetables

Calcium   Most green leafy vegetables

Iron   Spring greens, spinach, watercress and parsley

Potassium   Broccoli, spinach, green leafy vegetables

Yellow and orange fruit and vegetables

Vitamin A   Carrots, tomatoes, red peppers, apricots, mangoes, cantaloupe melons

Vitamin C   Oranges, lemons, grapefruit, kiwi fruit, mangoes, strawberries, blackberries, black-currants, cranberries, tomatoes, red and green peppers

Calcium   Blackcurrants and blackberries

speaking, dark or colourful fruit and vegetables contain more goodness than paler ones but they're all worth including so you get a good mix.

When is a legume not a vegetable?
When it's a peanut!

Believe it or not, the peanut is actually a legume, and studies show that about 25 g (1 oz) a day can be protective against heart disease and cancer. Although they are very similar to beans and pulses, they currently are not included in the five-a-day message, since their nutritional make-up is very different. Throw in a handful to enhance a stir-fry or salad, or whack some peanut butter and banana on bread for a tasty sandwich. Since, like most other nuts, they are lower in GiPs than you might expect, scattering a few on to your plate will help to lower the overall GI of the meal (unsalted nuts are best). Remember, though, that they are high in calories, so don't exceed 25 g/1 oz (a small handful) a day.

Hints and tips

● Eat five servings of fruit and vegetables every day. Remember that fruit juice can count as one of these servings but the GI will be higher.

● Buy fresh fruit and vegetables often and choose the highest quality that fits your budget, and ideally the firmest.

● Vegetables are generally low-GiP foods – aim to fill at least half your plate with them at main meals.

● Try to eat a salad or some fresh fruit at each meal. Skip salad dressings to keep the calories down, unless they're fat-free.

- Experiment with meals that are made up completely of raw food. You might enjoy the crunch and wholesomeness. Remember rainbow eating.

- Very often vitamins and minerals are concentrated just under the skin so scrub rather than peel potatoes, carrots and apples.

- Rather than leaving fruit or vegetables standing in water, where they lose more vitamin C, chop or slice them just before cooking.

- Go for frozen vegetables – they can often be fresher than fresh vegetables. Supermarket fresh vegetables are rarely picked the same day.

- Serve vegetables as soon as they're cooked.

Dairy products

This group includes milk, cheese, yoghurt and fromage frais. Dairy foods are excellent sources of calcium, and they also provide protein and vitamins. Calcium is vital for strong bones and teeth. Your bones are constantly being renewed and replaced, and right now you're probably not sitting on the same bones you were about seven years ago! Indeed children replace their skeleton roughly every two years. So you need a constant supply of bone-building nutrients to prevent your bones becoming weak in later life. Physical activity is also essential for strong bones. See Chapter 11 for tips on being more active.

Full-fat dairy foods can be high in saturated fat.

Too much of this type of fat may lead to raised blood-cholesterol levels, which in turn can increase your risk of heart problems. The GiP system takes this into account by offering you lower-saturated-fat versions of these foods. Aim for three different servings from this group each day to reach your recommended calcium levels. One serving is equivalent to 200 ml (⅓ pint) milk, one small pot of yoghurt or a small matchbox-size piece of cheese. Points have been allocated according to these serving sizes.

Vitamin D is needed to make use of the calcium in the foods you eat. Dairy products generally contain both vitamin D and calcium, so you get both nutrients at the same time. The body also makes vitamin D through the action of summer sunlight on the skin. Once made, vitamin D is stored in the liver for use during the winter.

Hints and tips

- Adults and children over five can choose skimmed or semi-skimmed milk in place of full-fat milk.
- Try low- or reduced-fat hard and soft cheeses. Check the labels to find those that are lowest. Medium-fat cheeses include Camembert, feta and mozzarella.
- Watch out for thick/creamy or Greek-style yoghurts which are higher in fat (but they are stilll better than cream).
- Choose a variety of dairy foods so that your three servings ideally come from different foods every day.

Meat, fish and alternatives

This group includes red meat, poultry, fish, eggs, pulses, Quorn, soya products (such as tofu), nuts and seeds. These foods are rich in protein and many are good sources of vitamins such as A and D, and minerals such as iron and zinc. Protein provides the building blocks for growth and repair of the body. In addition, most of the important chemicals in the body, including hormones such as insulin, are made of protein.

There is some research to show that protein foods reduce appetite, so you'll find that moderate amounts of protein are recommended in the GiP plan. Choosing home-cooked foods (such as grilled chicken breast), rather than a chicken ready meal (such as bought chicken casserole), will generally ensure that you get less salt and fewer additives. Too much protein can place a strain on the kidneys as they struggle to get rid of the waste products formed by the breakdown of protein. Choose 2–3 portions of protein foods a day, keeping to the amounts as suggested in the GiP table.

To reduce your saturated-fat intake, choose lean cuts of meat and minimise the fat you use in cooking. Processed meats such as burgers, pies, sausages and smoked meats tend to be higher in salt and fat, so aim to keep these foods to a minimum.

Opt for fish and vegetarian sources of protein as well as lean meats so that you get a variety. Vegetable proteins are also rich sources of fibre, vitamins such as folate, and antioxidants. You can make meat dishes healthier by adding beans or vegetables to recipes. This adds fibre, makes the meal go further and provides fewer calories per plate. What's more, since beans and vegetables tend to have a lower Glycaemic Index, adding them to casseroles and stews helps to keep your blood glucose steady, giving you energy for longer.

Oily fish

There is good evidence to show that oily fish can protect the heart, even in people with established heart disease. One of the most notable studies was the Diet and Reinfarction Trial, published in 1989, which studied 2,033 men under 70 years of age who had previously suffered a heart attack. One group increased their fish intake by eating 43 g (2 oz) of oily fish per day, which was three times higher than the other group. The results showed that there was a 29 per cent reduction in deaths, mostly those associated with coronary heart disease. In countries such as Japan, where people eat a lot of oily fish, the rates of heart disease are correspondingly low. Fish oil supplements have also been shown to have desirable effects on the heart.

The vital ingredient in oily fish is a fat called omega-3 and it is found in fish such as mackerel, herring, trout, tuna, salmon, sardines and pilchards. Current advice is to choose one portion of oily fish

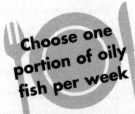

Choose one portion of oily fish per week

per week. Some eggs are now enriched with omega-3 fats, so if you're not a fish lover, this might be a helpful source for you. You also get some in soya beans, flaxseed and linseeds.

Hints and tips

- Select lean cuts of meat and trim off visible fat.
- Cook meat without adding fat. For example, grill, roast on a rack, microwave, barbecue, poach, dry-fry and braise.
- Avoid using the juices from roast meat for gravy.
- Remove the skin from poultry.
- Use spray-oil and a non-stick pan for stir-frying.
- If you're opting for vegetarian, remember that cheese and pastry can whack the fat up.
- Eat oily fish once a week.
- Nuts are an important source of protein if you are vegetarian. Recent research suggests that eating 25 g/1 oz (about a handful) of nuts such as almonds around five times a week may help protect against heart disease.
- Add canned beans or chick peas to soups and stews.
- If you are a curry addict, a dahl (lentil) curry is a tasty, healthy way to keep an eye on your GiPs. In takeaway meals, skim the oily layer from the top with a kitchen towel so you don't overdo the fat.
- Eat eggs poached, boiled or scrambled instead of fried. Limit to 5–6 eggs per week.

- If you rely on lots of convenience foods, look out for lower-fat and lower-salt versions of ready meals.
- Marinade and stir-fry some Quorn or tofu to help you choose low-fat protein foods.

Fatty and sugary foods

This group includes spreads, dressings, oils, crisps, pastries, rich sauces, sugar, confectionery, sugary drinks, jams, cakes and biscuits. Some fat provides essential fatty acids and vitamins. We even need some body fat for the protection and insulation of vital organs such as the heart and kidneys. However, we don't need all that much.

The whole issue of oils and fats can be confusing, for how can something be both bad and essential? We're told that high blood cholesterol is risky for the heart, yet foods high in cholesterol do not necessarily affect your blood cholesterol. Mediterranean eating gets the thumbs up, yet most of their salads swim in olive oil – how can this be?

In the Western world there is an abundance of fat-containing foods, and conditions such as obesity and heart disease are linked with a high-fat and high-calorie intake. So, boring though it may sound, moderation is always the key. Here are some home truths:

- Gram for gram, fat provides twice the calories of carbs or protein.

- Add fat and you bump up the calories. Fry an egg and the calories almost double, compared with a boiled or poached one.
- Fatty foods are often high in sugar too – think of Danish pastries and chocolate.
- Cooking oil has more fat and calories than butter, regardless of whether it's olive oil or corn oil.
- Some fats, such as omega-3, are essential and you need a regular supply from the food you eat. This is why foods like oily fish are so good for you.
- Your liver produces cholesterol irrespective of the cholesterol in your diet. So cholesterol from eggs and prawns, taken as part of a healthy diet, may have little effect on your blood cholesterol.
- You need fats to transport certain vitamins (fat-soluble ones) around the body.

Since we know that you will only lose weight if you take in fewer calories, it makes sense to limit the amount of fat that you eat. You'll notice that high-fat foods tend to have higher GiPs – this will encourage you to make healthier choices more often. Also, there is some evidence to show that calorie-dense foods such as burgers and chips tend to be less filling, so you are likely to over-eat. The GiP plan limits these and guides you towards low-GI and moderate-protein foods, which help to satisfy your appetite for longer.

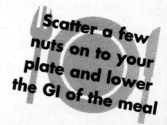

Scatter a few nuts on to your plate and lower the GI of the meal

Healthy eating isn't necessarily about low-fat – it's about the right fat, and balance.

People in Western countries generally eat far more fat than they need. You'll notice that some food labels offer guidance on how much fat you should aim for in a day. This works out at around 70 g fat per day for a woman and 95 g per day for a man.

In theory you could achieve your daily GiP target by choosing unwisely, for example eating mainly fatty foods. However, you would be breaking the GiP rules and not following the plan correctly. Also, this is unlikely to fill you up so you may end up actually eating more. As a result, you miss out on vital nutrients, become less healthy and may not lose weight. Therefore, as the GiP rules state, opt for a variety of low-GiP foods as often as you can as these will be inherently healthier. It is therefore a good idea to get into the habit of comparing food labels for their fat content, so you can make choices that fit into this target. For more on this, see Smart Shopping, Chapter 4.

So healthy eating isn't necessarily about low-fat – it's about the right fat. Research shows that a mono-unsaturated-fat-rich diet, as eaten in Mediterranean countries, may be preferable to a low-fat diet. Don't get too excited … This doesn't mean filling up on pies and sausages, because they do not contain the right types of fats for good health. Monounsaturates are found in foods like olive oil, rapeseed oil, almonds and other nuts, and avocados. Though high in fats, they

Fatty Swaps

Instead of ...	Try ...
Butter on bread	Grainy bread dipped in a little olive oil and balsamic vinegar
Corn oil in cooking	Rapeseed or olive oil
Sunflower oil in dressings	Fat-free dressings or a little walnut oil
Plain salad	Salad with a few added olives and walnuts
Rich desserts	Fruity puds or reduced-fat ice cream
Sugar-coated breakfast cereal	Muesli, porridge, wholegrain cereals
Mayonnaise	Low-fat yoghurt or fat-free dressings
Sugared fizzy drink	Unsweetened fruit juice, diet drink or water
Rich iced cake or doughnut	Fruit loaf, plain biscuits, oatmeal biscuits
Rich desserts	Low-fat fruit yoghurt, regular or reduced-calorie ice cream, fresh fruit, canned fruit in natural juice, sugar-free jelly, reduced-fat mousse

help you stay healthy and you may even lose weight in the right context. If you are a science addict, turn to page 338 for some research on this.

Since people who are overweight are at an increased risk of getting heart disease, watching your fat intake is particularly important. Eat less saturated fat, such as full-fat milk and cheese, fatty meat, lard, dripping, sausages, pies and pastries.

Replace some of the foods that contain a lot of saturated fat with those that are high in mono- or polyunsaturated fat. For example, use small amounts of rapeseed, olive, corn or sunflower oil in cooking, and a scraping of butter on bread, or choose a reduced-fat spread based on these oils. There is now a wide variety of lower-fat foods available in supermarkets. Use reduced-fat versions of dairy products, such as semi-skimmed or skimmed milk, half-fat Cheddar cheese and low-fat yoghurt. Note that reduced-fat doesn't mean no-fat – so don't go gorging on them just because the label says it's lower in fat.

The sweet stuff

Sugar, quite simply, can rot your teeth. If that's not a turn-off, then consider the fact that it can make you pile on the pounds. Since sweet foods tend to be high in fat as well (take chocolate or cakes for example), they are not a good choice for Gippers. Even more importantly, sugar in liquid form encourages your blood sugar to rise, so when you do want a sweet treat, think about the best time – such as after a low-GiP meal. As for how much, ask yourself what would be the minimum to help you curb that craving while still keeping to your GiP rules.

Fructose and lactose are types of sugar that are absorbed more slowly and so tend to avoid sugar rushes and energy highs and lows. You get fructose naturally from fruits, hence it is often called fruit sugar. You can now buy fructose in some supermarkets, and it is significantly lower in GI than ordinary sugar. Lactose comes from milk and milk products.

Sugar comes in many other guises. For example glucose, dextrose, maple syrup, golden syrup, honey, treacle, brown sugar, invert sugar, hydrolysed starch, and fruit juice. As with any ingredient, the higher up on the ingredients list an item appears, the more of it there is in the food.

If you would like to use a sugar substitute, artificial sweeteners such as saccharin, aspartame or acesulphame K are available in most supermarkets. They are much sweeter than sugar so much less can be used but some people find the taste off-putting. They are carbohydrate-free, so they don't raise your blood glucose. A new sweetener, sucralose (marketed as Splenda) is a sugar substitute that has been made from sugar. The GI is not available, but it has 2 calories per teaspoon (compared to 20 calories for sugar).

Hints and tips

● Swap fatty sauces and dressings for healthier options – try mixtures of lemon juice, vinegar, mustard or yoghurt and chuck in a few herbs and spices.

● Use healthier cooking methods such as grilling, baking, microwaving, poaching or stewing, instead of frying foods.

● Buy the leanest cuts of meat you can afford.

● Keep healthier titbits in your larder – the Snack Attack chapter (page 99) will have you oozing with ideas.

● Shop for monounsaturates, such as rapeseed oil, olive oil, nuts and seeds. And here's a bonus tip – rapeseed oil is much cheaper than olive oil, and is available in most supermarkets. Look closely at the label for rape-seed, as it is sometimes sold as vegetable oil.

● Consider bread without butter – do you really need it if you're going to be dipping the bread into soup, for example?

● Replace cream with half-fat crème fraîche, or Greek yoghurt.

● Eat fruit instead of sweets – the fructose in fruit is less damaging to your teeth and blood-glucose levels, compared to the sucrose in sweets.

● If you take sugar in tea or coffee, cut back half a teaspoon per cup each week. Your tastes have a strange way of adapting, so you'll find you do get used to it. Keep going and you'll cut out sugar altogether – better for the waistline and the teeth.

Salt

Salt is the common name for sodium chloride and it is the sodium part that is considered to be harmful if taken in excess. On a food label, you may not see salt on the ingredient list, but this doesn't mean that the food is sodium-free. Sodium can be listed in different ways, for example, monosodium glutamate, soy sauce, bicarbonate of soda and when a food is 'smoked'.

Good sense with salt is one of the key health messages, as eating too much salt has been associated with high blood pressure and strokes. If you eat too much salt it's likely that your body will hang on to excess water, which can lead to symptoms such as bloating, water retention and swollen ankles.

It is recommended that we eat no more than 6 g of salt (just over a teaspoon) a day. Yet, people in the UK probably get through at least 10 g or two teaspoons of salt each day. And the worst part is you probably don't even realise it. About two-thirds of the salt we consume comes from processed foods, such as bread, canned soups, breakfast cereals, sausages and savoury snacks. (Even sweet foods may contain salt.) So check the labels carefully. If most of the salt you eat comes from manufactured foods, and if you are addicted to ready meals and fast foods, you might be going overboard on the salt front.

Most food labels give you the amount of sodium, but the daily guidelines are based on the amount of

Salt content of some common foods

Food	Average sodium (grams)	Salt (grams)
Bread and cakes		
White bread – 1 medium slice	0.2	0.5
Wholemeal bread – 1 medium slice	0.2	0.5
1 Jam doughnut	negligible	0.1
1 Fruit scone	0.4	1.0
Biscuits		
1 Digestive biscuit	negligible	0.1
1 Chocolate digestive	negligible	0.2
1 Cream cracker	negligible	0.1
Cheeses		
Cheddar – small matchbox-size piece	0.2	0.5
Stilton – small matchbox-size piece	0.4	1.0
Cottage cheese – 2 tablespoons	0.4	1.0
Processed cheese – 2 slices	0.5	1.2
Meat, fish and eggs		
Bacon – 2 lean rashers	1.1	2.7
Sausages – 2 large	0.8	1.9
Ham – 1 lean slice	0.3	0.7
Roast chicken – 2 thick slices	negligible	0.2
1 Egg	negligible	0.2
Breakfast cereals		
2 Wheat biscuits	0.1	0.2
Cornflakes – medium bowl	0.3	0.7

Snacks		
Potato crisps – 25 g bag	0.2	0.5
Peanuts, salted – 50 g bag	0.2	0.5
Peanuts, dry roasted – 50 g bag	0.4	1.0
1 Banana	negligible	negligible
Vegetables		
Corn on the cob – average serving, unsalted	negligible	negligible
Sweetcorn – average serving, salted	0.3	0.7
Peas – average serving, salted	negligible	0.2
Pasta		
Spaghetti in tomato sauce – ½ standard can	1.0	2.4
Macaroni cheese – 5 tablespoons	0.7	1.7

salt. So, to work out the amount of salt in a food, you simply multiply the sodium figure by 2.5 (2.4 to be precise!). And since this is often per 100 g of the food, you then need to work out how much salt you get in a portion if the label doesn't tell you. Easy? Hmmm … We've done some of the working out for you (see table opposite) so you can compare some common foods.

Hints and tips

● Processed, convenience foods are often loaded with salt. These include sausages, bacon, savoury pastries, some canned fish and smoked foods such as smoked fish. Instead choose fresh fish, meat, fruit and vegetables. Only a small amount of salt is present naturally.

● Cut down on salty foods such as crisps, savoury biscuits and salted nuts. Choose fresh fruit, unsalted nuts and dried fruit as alternative snacks.

● Think about the amount of salt you add in cooking and gradually use less.

● Avoid adding salt at the table.

● Experiment with new flavours such as exotic herbs, freshly ground spices, freshly ground black pepper and paprika. Also try lime juice, balsamic vinegar and chilli sauce. If you find it hard to adjust to less salt, try a salt substitute, which enhances the flavour without adding so much sodium. Low-salt products (such as tuna in water, canned vegetables in water, unsalted bread and butter) are available in supermarkets and can be used instead of salt-rich foods.

Water

Did you know that around 60 per cent of your body weight is water? We continually need to replace the amount we lose each day in our breath, sweat and urine. You need even more fluid if you're in a centrally heated or air-conditioned environment.

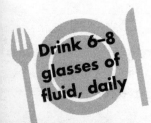
Drink 6–8 glasses of fluid, daily

Drink at least 1.5 litres/3 pints (6–8 glasses) of fluid each day. Some people find that keeping a bottle of water on their desk makes this easier, especially as seeing water may make you more conscious of your thirst. However, you needn't restrict yourself to plain water. Have a variety of drinks, such as unsweetened fruit juice, sugar-free soft drinks, lower-fat milk and flavoured waters. You may have a few cups of tea and coffee, too, if you like.

Many soft drinks, including fruit juice, contain sugar and this raises their Glycaemic Index. So drinking large amounts of fruit juice, even if unsweetened, may make your blood glucose rise sharply. This is because sugar in liquid form is rapidly absorbed by the body. If you like fresh fruit juice, drink it with a meal rather than on its own. Tomato juice is particularly low in GiPs, so choose it in preference to higher-GiP sweetened drinks. Be particularly cautious with high-energy glucose drinks – they send your blood glucose up very quickly and hence are higher in GiPs.

An easy way to check if you're drinking enough is to look at the colour of your urine the next time you go to the loo. If it's pale and there's lots of it, then you're probably drinking enough. If you're passing less urine and it's darker, then this could be a sign of dehydration.

Mediterranean olive groves and orchards

Fed up of the same old messages – eat less fat, eat more fibre and eat less sugar? Then here's a lifestyle that'll really tickle your taste buds. The Mediterranean way of eating, with an abundance of olive oil, fish, nuts, fruit and veggies, has been associated with a lower risk of conditions such as coronary heart disease and cancer. Interestingly, the total amount of fat eaten by people who live in Mediterranean countries is actually quite high. But take a closer look and you'll see that it's high in monounsaturated fats (such as olive oil) and omega-3 fats (such as those found in oily fish). Studies on 'Med-eating' support the idea that opting for the right types of fat may be more important than getting your fat intake really low.

Research suggests that as little as 25 g (1 oz) of oily fish a day can significantly lower the incidence of heart disease. People in these countries also have a much higher intake of fruit and vegetables, so they benefit from a good antioxidant intake. They eat more garlic, and this characteristic ingredient of Mediterranean cuisine also has therapeutic properties. Garlic has been shown to thin the blood, helping it to flow more smoothly. Garlic also contains the natural antibiotic allicin.

Study after study has shown that nuts such as walnuts, almonds and peanuts, commonly consumed in the Mediterranean countries, are beneficial to

Acting out of well-informed choices today will shape your life tomorrow.

health. Rich in monounsaturated fats, they are, however, high in calories, so keep to a small handful (about 25 g or 1 oz) a day, especially if you're watching your waistline.

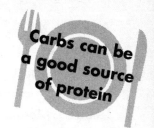

Carbs can be a good source of protein

Taking a leaf from the olive tree, it makes sense to incorporate the healthy aspects of Mediterranean cuisine into a balanced slimming plan. So, enjoy the Mediterranean musts – garlic, fruit and veg, fish, a glass of red wine (see next chapter), beans and lentils, a handful of nuts and taking your time over your meal.

Supplements – who needs them?

It is preferable to get our nutrients from natural foods where possible. However, we do live in the real world, with hectic lifestyles, stress, and the availability of ready meals and takeaways. It's not always easy to eat well. You might therefore want to take an all-round supplement as a safety net, but do ensure it provides no more than 100 per cent of the recommended daily amount (RDA) of particular vitamins and minerals. If you are tempted by supplements that offer large doses of vitamins or minerals, proceed with caution. Some of these nutrients are stored by the body and can be harmful if taken in excess.

Certain groups, such as pregnant women and the elderly, may require particular supplements and are advised to speak to their doctor.

Are you a Real Gipper?

Question:

When you're watching your weight, what do you do?

Choice 1: Mostly, I eat regularly and in small amounts and I aim for a slow, steady weight loss. I really only eat when I'm hungry.

A weight loss of ½–1 kg (1–2 lb) per week is the best way to ensure that the weight stays off! Eating six times a day is ideal for the 'Gipper'.

Choice 2: I'm currently making gradual changes to my lifestyle – healthy foods and regular exercise.

A tailored approach is great – the sure way to becoming slimmer is to choose a plan that fits in with your current lifestyle. Team this up with regular physical activity and you've got it made!

Choice 3: I often try crash diets and milk-shake diets as they promise quick results!

There is no healthy way to lose weight fast. Such diets encourage a dieting mentality and yo-yo dieting is more harmful to your health than being slightly overweight.

Results:

Choice 1: You'll appreciate a state of consistent high energy and a sense of overall well-being that will help you to sustain a positive mental attitude. This is likely

to support you in reaching/maintaining your ultimate weight.

Choice 2: You've done the trickiest part! You're
making important changes, today. The choices that
you make now will shape your life.

Choice 3: Change your thinking so that achieving
your goal becomes pleasurable and fun. Let it become
an enticing way of enriching your life. This way,
you're likely to succeed long term, as opposed to
quick-fix methods that don't necessarily last!

**So be a Real Gipper – and choose in line with the
new you.**

Summary
- The more varied the colours on your plate, the more
  varied the nutrients.
- Porridge and muesli are ideal in GiP-eating, as are
  pulses: choose them regularly.
- Most fruit and veg are low in points: include five, daily.

10

ALCOHOL – FRIEND OR ENEMY?

Sensible drinking

You may feel that choosing a healthy lifestyle means your days of having a drink at the pub or a glass of wine over dinner will be numbered. Our general philosophy is nothing is out of bounds. The key is balance, and making the right choices for you. Today's choices become tomorrow's consequences. And, should you indulge in two or three drinks too many, you can count on your body letting you know, in no uncertain terms!

Know your units

There's no reason why you cannot enjoy a drink (unless of course you have been advised to avoid alcohol for medical reasons), so long as you make sensible choices and drink in moderation. On the GiP programme, the ideal amount is no more than 7 units per week for a woman, and 10 units for a man. Alcohol does add calories, some drinks more than others, so the less you drink, the better for your target weight.

1 unit of alcohol = ½ pint beer or lager = 1 standard glass of wine = 1 pub measure of spirits, sherry, aperitif or liqueur.

Follow these guidelines:

Use calorie-free mixers

- Avoid drinking on an empty stomach.
- Wherever possible, intersperse your alcoholic drinks with water or soft drinks.
- If you enjoy spirits, mix single measures with sugar-free or low-calorie mixers.
- Avoid alcopops and creamy cocktails.

Pub measures have become more generous, so take care you are not consuming more units than you think, especially if the bartender is a friend! Here are the average units in some popular pub-measure tipples:

- A glass of champagne – 2 units
- A glass of wine – 2 units
- Bottle of beer – 1.5 units
- Pint of lager – 2 units
- Vodka and Red Bull – 1 unit

Weighty matters

Weight for weight, alcohol contains more calories than sugar, so even moderate drinking can make you gain weight. For example, one pint of beer has around the same calories as three chocolate biscuits. Replacing meals with alcoholic drinks can mean that you lose out on important vitamins and minerals, so it's simply a matter of thinking about how much you drink and when.

Excessive drinking, whether it is every day or one session a week (binge drinking) can lead to long-term effects such as tremors, memory loss, heart disease, stomach ulcers and cancer. Also, it can cause your bones to thin, as you don't absorb nutrients so effectively. It is also known to trigger sudden drops in blood-sugar levels, which is especially important if you have diabetes.

And now for the silver lining!

Moderate drinking can be good for you. Red wine in moderation has been shown to increase levels of good cholesterol in the blood. It may also prevent blood

> A thousand-mile journey starts with one small step. *(Lao-tse)*

clots because of its blood-thinning properties. The active ingredients in red wine are phenols. These act in a similar way to the antioxidant vitamins in fruit. Taken together, these properties mean red wine may help protect against heart disease. Therefore one glass of red wine a day can be beneficial to health, as part of a balanced lifestyle.

Hitting the pause button

Ask yourself, 'Why do I really want that drink?' Drinking is commonly associated with the need to feel more relaxed, especially in social circumstances. What need does it meet in your case that is not being met in any other way? Once you have identified this, you can start to find creative ways to meet that need – without the excessive drinking. For some people alcohol is a comfort blanket. If you are in this category, hit the pause button, *before* you reach for that next drink. Pause long enough to ask yourself whether this is what you really choose for yourself and how it may be affecting others in your life who are important to you.

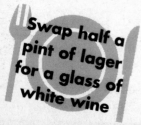
Swap half a pint of lager for a glass of white wine

The only thing I cannot resist is temptation!

For many, drinking excessively is a habit – a case of having something in your hand. And, like any habitual pattern, it **can** be broken. So, for example, make a conscious effort to distract yourself by moving around. Any change in your body movements will have an influence on your thinking. Consider going for a walk, or choose another form of exercise that you enjoy. Take a bath, clear your desk, read a book or make a phone call. If you're in a pub, have a game of pool or darts. The chances are that if or when the thought of a drink returns, it will do so with less temptation, so that you are more likely to let it go.

Be positive

The mind is a powerful tool and its strength can be used to make healthy changes to everyday aspects of your life, including your drinking habits. As you think it, so shall you be.

Change the way you talk to yourself by switching from negative to positive language and focusing your

By refocusing towards what it is that you'd really like, you are likely to get the results that you really choose.

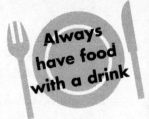

Always have food with a drink

thoughts in a different direction. If you can break patterns, you can deal with anything! If you break a pattern often enough it will eventually disappear. For example, if you catch yourself saying, 'I'm hopeless at resisting another pint', you could change this to: 'When I put my mind to it, I am determined to stay focused on getting a flatter belly.' Practise saying the kinds of things that are positively reinforcing and encouraging.

Summary
- Weekly allowance = 7 units for women, 10 units for men. This is in addition to your daily points total.
- Have two or three alcohol-free days each week.
- Distract yourself before you reach for a tipple too many!

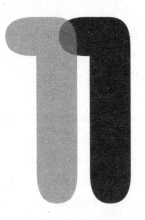

GET
PHYSICAL

Shift your bun and lose a ton!

Is this you?
- Every day you look in the mirror and say, 'If I lose a few pounds, I'll be happier, successful, more attractive ...'
- You lose weight but you are still unhappy, because inside you still think of yourself as being fat.

The human body is the best picture of the human soul. *(Ludwig Wittgenstein)*

● You are overweight, feel unhappy and are finding it hard to break the cycle of yo-yo dieting and/or other unhealthy eating patterns.

The Gi Point Diet recommends short chunks of regular physical activity that are easy to fit into your daily routine. Being physically active while taking part in any weight-loss programme is integral to long-term success. If you can maintain some sort of regular activity (and this could be as simple as taking the dog for a brisk walk), it can help you keep the weight off once you reach your target. For exercise to be of lasting benefit, make it as regular as brushing your teeth and take it as seriously as your driving test.

Exercise is often linked with a healthy self-image and can become a positive addiction! When you make up your mind to commit to getting fitter, so that it becomes second nature, the chances are that you'll start to love it and to look forward to it. The key is to choose an activity you enjoy and that fits in with your lifestyle. When you get it right, you're likely to find that it produces more and more pleasure and you begin to experience a newfound level of vitality and energy that, up to now, you may only have dreamt of.

Create the energy to exercise just by going for it. Too much thinking can slow you down! If much of your day is spent behind a desk, or in a stuffy environment, you may well feel lethargic and tired. In that case moving around and getting some fresh air will have an even greater and more beneficial impact. Think about doing some physical activity as soon as you finish work or once you get home. Just 10 minutes can make a big difference.

Self-image

When you're not feeling great about yourself, it shows and 'leaks' out in so many ways. This can be conscious or unconscious. For example, you may suffer more illness, or binge out on food, alcohol or drugs. You are reinforcing that you don't deserve to be happy. As your behaviour comes from your thoughts, you proceed to live out this image, continually finding ways to prove it to be true! It turns into a self-fulfilling prophecy and you'll find yourself in various situations and relationships that will reaffirm this. People treat you the way you treat yourself. So, develop a healthy self-love and you're likely to develop a kinder, more caring attitude towards your health and, in turn, your body.

If you dislike your body, here's what you can do:

● Be mindful that your behaviour is consistent with who you think you are.
● Change the way you think and talk *about* yourself and *to* yourself. Your happiness depends on it. Say only positive things, or nothing at all! Think of

words or phrases that you enjoy hearing and repeat them to yourself throughout the day.

- Your thoughts are revealed through your physiology. By examining your body today you'll know how you were thinking all the yesterdays that have been and gone. If you want to know what you'll look like tomorrow, examine your thinking today. Change your thoughts and you change your reality.

- Picture yourself as being exactly the way you want to be. The best way to become who you most want to be is to act as if you have already become that person, today. Fake it till you make it!

Ways to boost your self-esteem

- Recognise your own value as successful people do by saying 'thank you', when you're given a compliment – and then shut up! When a friend tells you that you look 'hot', accept their gift without responding, 'Yes, but I've got huge thighs!'

- Form relationships with those who treat you with respect.

- Compliment others and mean it.

- Praise yourself by acknowledging your worth – and mean it!

- Separate your behaviour from your identity. If you do or say something stupid, it doesn't make you a stupid person.

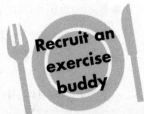

Recruit an exercise buddy

- Treat your body well through exercise and a healthy diet.
- Set examples to others by how you treat yourself.
- Surround yourself with great people.
- See yourself as you want to be daily and act as if you're already it.
- Inspire yourself with health books and workshops.

Health and fitness are not the same. Fitness is about the ability to perform physical activity. Health can be defined as the state in which all the systems of the body are working optimally. Ideally, you will wish for both. By putting health first, you will promote great benefits in your life. Society has changed over the decades. Previously, daily life involved accomplishing chores in a physical way. Now, we are at the mercy of PCs and mobiles – we don't even need to walk to the telephone booth!

If you're normally inactive and are now really serious about building up your stamina and fitness levels, it's best to *seek advice from your GP*. Taking responsibility for your own training schedule is not everyone's cuppa and is perhaps easier for those who are naturally motivated and self-disciplined. Even if you are, you will want to build up your knowledge and potential safely, with the support of a fitness instructor, working with an optimal programme that will produce the best results. Recruiting an exercise buddy can be a great motivator, too. By exercising with a friend you're much more likely to coax and cheer each other on, turn up even when you'd rather not, and have some great laughs along the way, especially when you choose something that you both really enjoy.

Use it or lose it

Whatever you don't use, you lose. It's easy to see this in your physical body. If you decided to spend a year in an armchair for no reason other than that you liked sitting down, once the year was up you probably wouldn't be able to walk. If you stop using your legs they will stop working! Moving around and exercising is great news for your body, for example, as it helps to build up your bones. It enhances the performance of your brain, too. But you also have to use your mind to keep that in shape. Use your mental capacity to the full as the years go by and it will continue to work for you. As with exercising, practise stretching your mind by extending your creative imagination. A simple and fun way is to become more creative with your healthy food choices and daily menu planning (while remaining within the GiP system). Making the most of what you *do* have means you get to keep it!

Fit for a king or queen

Remote controls, cordless phones and internet shopping are only a few of the devices that are bringing us closer to becoming a nation of couch potatoes. And with that comes an increased risk of obesity, and all the nasty disorders associated with it. Keeping fit is one of the best preventive medicines available to you, often at no extra cost. Whatever your age, a total of 30 minutes of moderate exercise five times a week is a great insurance policy. It can be as simple as a brisk walk divided into three 10-minute chunks. This equates to around 150 minutes of 10-minute slots each week. The Gi Point Diet recommends two 10-minute bursts a day (see page 204), which is around 140 minutes per week. Try these:

- Walk further to buy your lunch.
- Get off the bus or train a stop before you need to and walk the rest of the way.
- Use the stairs when you can – ups are better than downs!
- Walk up *and* down escalators.
- Dance to your favourite music around the home: you could combine it with doing your daily chores. Even 30 minutes of slow dancing knocks off the cals.
- Try gardening and various forms of DIY.
- Spend quality time with the children in a swimming pool or the park. This can be an energetic and fun way to engage with your kids.
- Walk the dog, or borrow a neighbour's! It's also a great way to make new friends.
- Play golf. It is an excellent way to drum up new business – work and play all rolled into one.

Get GiP-fit

Whatever your daily activity levels, congratulate yourself that you're doing something. Add to this whatever activity you feel you can perform comfortably and happily. Every little bit helps. You don't need to exercise for half an hour at a time to get the benefit – being GiP-fit means only doing two 10-minute bursts of reasonably brisk physical activity daily. Add this to your current daily routine and you're making a big difference to your fitness and activity levels.

Being active doesn't mean you have to do planned 'exercise' in the form of a class or the gym. But if you do, that's great! Remember that just getting off that chair and moving can have an impact. And if you make moving a habit, it will help you feel less lethargic. Make your 10-minute bursts planned sessions, and aim to feel slightly breathless and warm as you exercise.

Shedding those pounds is a simple balance between the calories you take in as food and the calories you use up by daily physical activity. Eating fewer calories will help you shift those unwanted bulges. Incorporating regular activity helps to mobilise your fat stores, and burn calories, so you lose

GiP Rule 7:
Have at least two 10-minute bursts of moderate-intensity physical activity every day.

Chart your activity progress

Use this chart to record how many of the 10-minute activity sessions you're taking each day. Simply pencil in a tick every time, aiming for two ticks per day.

	Mon	Tue	Wed	Thur	Fri	Sat	Sun
Week 1							
Week 2							
Week 3							
Week 4							
Week 5							
Week 6							

weight even more effectively. And if you keep up the GiP programme, you're more likely to stay trim and fit for longer.

Feeling hot, hot, hot!

Here are some quickies to get you started whether you're at home, in the office, car or bedroom. Yes, it is possible to burn off the cals and tone up without too much effort. The recipe to continued success is making exercise a part of your daily routine. Getting to a swimming pool can be hard work, as can going to the gym, regularly. But there's lots of other things you can do. Get off those buns and get going! Here's how.

The home

- Gardening – you can burn off around 150 calories in half an hour of applying yourself to some spade work, for example.
- Running up and down stairs 10 times a day will eat up around 250 calories as well as helping you to tone those thighs and the derrière.
- Ironing alone can shift up to 150 calories in half an hour and vacuuming for around 30 minutes can help you lose another 200.

Household chores may no longer be a chore!

The office

- Park the car 10 minutes away or at the other end of the car park. A brisk walk to the office will help you to burn off those cals.
- Instead of sending another dreaded e-mail, walk over to your colleague's desk.
- Ditch the lift and take the stairs – two at a time when the need arises.

The car

- At the superstore, park as far away as you can from the entrance. Leave the trolley by the store so that you have to carry your bags back to the car, toning up along the way.
- If you're a parent, consider walking

Household chores may no longer be a chore!

the kids to school instead of taking the car. You'll be less stressed, through avoiding the rush-hour congestion, and your children are likely to be more

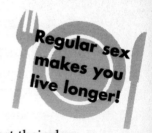

Regular sex makes you live longer!

energised and alert when they start their day.

- Have you thought about buying a bike? One hour of cycling will help shift around 330 calories and it will strengthen your lungs, heart, legs and back. Set aside the money that you save on petrol and reward yourself in some way.

The bedroom

It's free and you'll burn off plenty of calories, too! Just 30 minutes of sexy-cise will burn off around 200 cals. Sex is also said to lift your mood, reduce stress and boost your circulation. It's great for toning stomach and inner thighs. And if this fun, fitness and frivolity isn't enough, research tells us that regular sex makes you live longer.

All the activities suggested here will help you shift those stubborn calories, but the amounts given can only be a guide as everyone is unique.

Find a form of exercise that you love and enjoy and build it into your daily routine.

Beat the blues

Interestingly, there is a strong link between exercise and mental health. People who choose regular exercise are less likely to suffer depression, by keeping themselves more uplifted and motivated. Waking up daily with a fresh feeling of optimism and enthusiasm is just what any doctor would prescribe, on tap! This is important when you are setting about achieving your outcome of becoming the new you. Those who do experience depression can reduce their symptoms through regular exercise. Its effect is immediate and long-lasting, as the body's natural pharmacy releases mood-enhancing chemicals. Regular exercise also reduces the likelihood of depression returning. The link between the mind and body is inextricable because the chemicals that exercise produces promote well-being.

Horsey tale

Once upon a time there lived a king who, as all dads do, doted upon his two daughters. Most subjects within the kingdom couldn't tell the young girls apart, except when they spoke. One was the eternal optimist, whereas her sister was the eternal pessimist. Of course, this difference was a hot topic of gossip in the grounds. However, the doting father refused to believe it and decided once and for all to put it to the test. So, one Christmas, he crept into their rooms and left their presents. For the pessimist, he had filled a stocking so that it was brimming with many colourful and dazzling packages of the most exquisite gifts. For the optimist, he simply shovelled huge amounts of horse manure into her room as she lay soundly asleep. As dawn broke, he heard the stirring from his daughters' rooms and decided to risk a peek. To his astonishment, the pessimist was moaning about not wanting any of the gifts and what a disappointment the whole Christmas thing turned out to be, time and time again. Also to his amazement, when he listened at the optimist's door, he could hear non-stop giggles, and when he opened it, the sight of her shovelling the horse manure out of her window greeted him. 'What makes you so happy?' he asked her. She replied, in between the laughter, 'With this amount of horse manure, there must be a pony hiding somewhere!'

Float your boat

Imagine yourself as vividly as you can, being the new you in every which way. See yourself incorporating exercise into your everyday routine and see how effortlessly it fits in with your lifestyle. Be specific in how you are being active and for how long. Consider all areas of your life. What changes, even small ones, are you making as you go about your life in the home, work, car, bedroom, gym and anywhere else? In the absence of a personal trainer, you can learn how to become highly motivated and inspirational to yourself, not to mention others along the way.

Give yourself feedback

If what you are doing isn't working or has stopped working, then try something else. Be specific about your weight loss, if that is your goal, by determining exactly how much weight you want to lose by a certain date. Write this down. Share your goal with others. They can then challenge and support you along the way. You never know, they may even join in. Make it a biggie. By the end of a realistic time period, see yourself doing something highly motivational, for example, running a marathon, doing a sponsored bike ride or a charity swim, whatever floats your boat! Most importantly, enjoy yourself along the way.

Do try this at home!

Make a commitment to yourself. You are the most important product of your life. By looking after yourself, you ensure you will be there for others. Develop your lifestyle plan by aiming for simple bite-size chunks. This way, you're more likely to over-achieve. You'll feel great, and your motivation will reach a momentum all of its own, as you know you can do it! Take a moment to think about what is truly important to you.

Consider how you can commit to make the following changes in your life.

Give yourself a score between 1 and 10, 1 being the lowest.

	now	in the future	by when
1 Your diet			

Think in terms of a balanced nutritious diet.

	now	in the future	by when
2 Fitness			

Think in terms of how much physical activity you are getting. Include examples such as gardening, walking, and climbing stairs.

	now	in the future	by when
3 Sports			

Do you play any sports?

	now	in the future	by when
4 Other			

How do you nourish your physical being (for example, through reflexology, massage, other types of treatment)?

How will achieving these changes make your life different? Consider making a list. This will bring the answers to the forefront of your mind. Act on them!

There are many, many reasons for making regular exercise a natural part of your daily routine. Here are some reminders about the benefits of exercise:

- Improves muscular strength and increases flexibility.
- Helps prevent varicose veins.
- Enhances your posture.
- Aids lower back pain and strengthens the spine.
- Helps to reduce anxiety, tension and stress.
- Enhances self-esteem and confidence.
- Helps prevent premature ageing.
- Supports a balanced and healthy diet.
- Helps to beat the blues.
- Helps to keep up a healthy body image and good sex life.
- Burns calories.
- Reduces the risk of heart disease, osteoporosis and cancer.

Your body acts as your mirror

And much more!

Behind the desk

Is this you? You sit in a car or on a bus or train on your way to work. You then sit behind a desk for eight hours before heading home. You reward yourself by falling into a comfy armchair and pretty much staying there for the evening! Of course, there's always a pay-off in remaining just as you are.

Being a couch potato gives you something of value. If it didn't, you would have made the change already! Facing up to what the unmet need is is a milestone in your thinking. It is only by acknowledging this that you can then begin to build it into your ultimate goal, so that the perceived value that it gives you is replaced in a healthier and more functional way. For example, an elderly relative who constantly complains about her illnesses may (unconsciously) think that this brings her more visits from her family. But if she were to stop complaining, the regularity of the visits might increase. Unless and until she realises that the visits would increase because her new cheery disposition is likely to attract more, she may well remain as she is.

If you recognise yourself here, then this chapter's definitely for you. And, even if your life isn't sedentary, you'll find some very useful stuff anyway!

Think like an active person

Thinking like an active person will send the relevant message to your brain to act like one. It will make you feel more positive and help you deal resourcefully with the challenges of the day ahead. To inspire you even more, how about putting up an 'ideal new you' picture to spur you on. When you are feeling motivated, you can conquer Everest (almost)!

Behind the desk – get physical at every opportunity!

● Instead of sending e-mails or making internal telephone calls, walk over to the other end of the building, visit a different floor, leave your seat and talk to the person, face to face. Not only will this stretch your body, use up calories, raise your activity levels and boost your energy a tad, the personal touch promotes rapport with your colleagues.

- When you go to buy lunch, choose somewhere a little further away.
- Drinking plenty of water during the day is a must, so take regular walks to the water cooler or kitchen, throughout the day. This will help you use up the calories as well as keeping you hydrated.
- Work on your feet! You'll burn calories by standing up and make your brain more alert. Do this hourly for several minutes at a time.

Remember that planned snacks make good sense. Go for low-GI snacks such as apples, dried apricots and pears. For a host of quick and easy snack ideas at the office, turn to page 102.

Keyboard yoga – hand and wrist

Important! Before you begin

If the thought of breathing lessons sounds too boring for words, just remember to breathe deeply. When doing the following exercises take it all in and let it all out. Breathing is good for you! Breathe deeply into your abdomen, as this is a great way to oxygenate your body, especially when you're tense.

After completing this fun and funky yoga at your desk, it's a good idea to drink plenty of water. While you may not feel thirsty, your body will thank you.

Hands in prayer pose

1 Sit with your back straight and both feet flat on the floor. Place your hands together, finger-to-finger, palm-to-palm, in prayer pose in front of your heart.

2 Slowly inhale, pressing the palms of your hands firmly together, fingers pointing up. Holding the prayer pose, exhale slowly as you lower your hands as far as possible.

3 Maintaining the prayer pose, inhale and slowly raise your hands in front of your heart. Then, exhale slowly and lower your hands. Repeat, five to 10 times.

4 To complete this posture: inhale, keeping your hands in front of your chest, then exhale, relaxing your chin to your chest.

Counter-stretch for prayer pose

1 Sit with your back straight and both feet flat on the floor. Stretch your arms out in front of your chest with your shoulders relaxed, palms together and fingers interlaced.

2 Reach outwards with your arms and hands, keeping your back straight. Inhale slowly, raising your arms above the crown of your head. Allow your entire spine to stretch tall and long.

3 Exhale slowly, feeling the length of your spine, and

return your hands to their position in front of your heart. Repeat, five to 10 times.

4 To complete this posture: inhale, pressing your palms up to the sky, then exhale, slowly allowing your hands to float down to your sides.

Source: www.ivillage.co.uk

Armchair exercises

Your body exists now as a result of the choices you have made through your life, in the past, up to this point, today. Your body acts as your mirror. If you look at your physiology today, you know how you were thinking all the yesterdays. So, if in your thinking you were content enough to be a couch potato, your physiology will resemble this. If you want to know how you will look tomorrow, examine your thinking today! Your 'temple' has acted as a field of all your thoughts and ideas and can be transformed in the physical sense if you are willing to change your ideas. In other words if you don't like what you've chosen, choose again. The mind and body are inextricably linked. Celebrate the choices that you have made, knowing that you can choose to take some significant learning from them. This is empowering and highly motivating. And, how about this? You

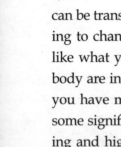
Exercise in your armchair

can do something about this even when you're in the comfy chair!

It is advisable to consult with your doctor before starting any new exercise regime especially if you are normally inactive, and these exercises are no exception.

To tighten and lift the buttock muscles

1 Make sure you are sitting comfortably.
2 Squeeze the buttocks together as tightly as possible.
3 Hold the squeeze for a slow count of three.

Aim to do this at least 10 times to start with, more if you can manage it – the more you do, the tighter your bottom will become! If you are squeezing hard, you should feel yourself 'lift' slightly.

To flatten and tone the tummy muscles

1 Sitting comfortably, lean forward slightly, placing the hands on the thighs. Take a deep breath in through the nose.
2 Breathing out through the mouth, pull the tummy muscles in tightly (imagine you are trying to get your navel to touch your spine). Hold the position for a few seconds, breathing normally.
3 Relax and take another breath in through the nostrils.
4 Breathe out through the mouth and repeat, pulling in the tummy muscles.

Do this exercise five times to start with, gradually increasing the repetitions as you build up strength. It is a good way of toning and flattening the abdominal muscles, so persevere!

Convert your inner thoughts into outer energy.
Become who you most wish to be.

To strengthen the chest muscles

This exercise improves the appearance of the bust. In men, it firms up flabby tissue and develops 'firm pecs' (pectoral muscles).

1 Sitting up straight, bring the arms up and bend the elbows. Press the palms of the hands together in the 'praying' position (keep the elbows high and out to the sides).
2 Squeeze the heels of the hands together as firmly as possible. You should feel the pectoral muscle (under the arms and to the sides of the chest) working.

Aim to do 30 repetitions to start with at a pace of one squeeze per second. When you can do this comfortably, do an additional set of 15, holding the squeeze for a slow count of three. Release and repeat.

These exercises are taken from *Rosie's Armchair Exercises* by Rosita Evans, published by Discovery Books, 29 Hacketts Lane, Woking GU22 8PP (01932 400800). For further fab, beat the flab exercises you can do from the comfort of your home send for a copy – just £5.99, including p&p.

Stillness of breath

Breathing is a natural instinct, although breathing properly may not be. Breathing oxygenates the blood and is a mirror to our physical and emotional state. Mastering simple breathing techniques can do wonders to de-stress and ease tensions and aches.

During the day, find time for a few precious minutes of peaceful time by trying out this simple yet effective calming and rejuvenating breathing exercise. It will relax you in body and mind.

1 Sit with your back straight and close your eyes. Take a deep breath and push your tummy out like an inflated balloon.

2 Let your breath out accompanied by the sound of 'om' (you could make this sound almost silently, if you choose), simultaneously drawing your tummy into your spine. An alternative is to concentrate your breathing through your nose.

3 Allow your breathing to find its natural rhythm, calming your mind by focusing on each breath. If your mind wanders, simply redirect it and carry on.

Summary

- Keeping fit is one of the best preventive medicines.
- Regular exercise helps keep the blues at bay.
- Have at least two 10-minute bursts of brisk but sustainable physical activity every day.
- Deep breathing will relax you in body and mind.
- Leading a sedentary lifestyle gives you something of value. What is the unmet need in you?
- Be prepared and have low-GI snacks in your desk drawer, ready for that energising break.

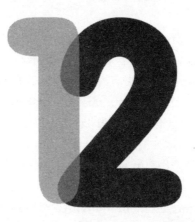

12

GET YOUR
MIND ON
YOUR SIDE

Switch your thinking

In June 2002 the Diabetes Research and Wellness Foundation launched 'Think Well To Be Well', a new concept in caring for people with diabetes. As 70–80 per cent of diabetics are overweight, the concept is

Whatever you can do, or dream you can ... begin it. Boldness has genius, power and magic in it. *(Goethe)*

especially appropriate for anyone wanting to lose a few pounds. Bringing a fresh approach to diet, the concept helps people to take control of their lives and to focus on achieving sustainable results. The Gi Point Diet embraces the 'Think Well' philosophy and it is this – and more – that we bring you in this book.

Even with the most effective dietary advice, your new way of eating might be short-lived unless you have prepared yourself mentally with a resourceful and positive mental approach. After all, if you follow the same way of thinking wherever you go, regardless of the environment, situation, or relationship you are in, nothing changes, because you haven't made any adjustment to your thoughts. Some people believe that if only they lived in a bigger house, drove a smarter car, got a promotion, owned a holiday beach home in Barbados, changed their partner, their kids and their dog, their lives would be sorted and they would be blissfully happy. Not so! Without a fundamental switch in their thinking, it would simply be same old, same old …

For the Gi Point Diet – indeed any lifestyle change – to be really effective, there are some key things to think about. You have chosen to look at this book *right now*, for whatever reason. By doing that, you have

If you always do what you have always done, you will always get what you always got.

Knowledge is not enough unless it is supported by a positive approach and mental attitude. By changing your thoughts you change your world, through choosing different actions.

transferred a thought (such as 'I need to lose weight') into action by picking up the book and flicking through its pages. You have just demonstrated an important principle: everything we do starts from a thought, which then has the potential to spur us into action.

Everything that exists does so because it started as a seed, an idea, in someone's mind. We know, of course, that the mind is an extremely powerful tool, and one that we understand and use so little. So the first step to successful dieting is looking at what's going on in that brain of yours.

Many scientists would refer to the strategies in this book as cognitive behavioural therapy, neuro-linguistic programming and psychology. Couple this with strong evidence of nutritional science and dietetics, and you have a broad, balanced range of expertise.

The thinking body

You are what you think. As you think it, so you become it. You can only act out of your thoughts. For example, you have the choice to pick up the juicy apple or the chocolate bun. Where does that action come from? Your thoughts, of course!

The mind–body link is an inseparable unit. Making a change in one area automatically affects the other.

Deciding how you shape your health, including the choices that you make relating to eating habits, is key to your well-being. Thinking happy and healthy thoughts will influence your health, feelings and emotions and they will also be revealed – quite literally – in your body. Your mind is a phenomenal tool. Try this:

Acting like a lemon!

Think of a lemon. See it in front of you and make the image as real and bright as you can. See its colour, clearly, and picture the small uneven grooves in the skin. Now, in your mind's eye, run your finger along it, feeling the texture of its skin. With a knife, cut it in half. See the two halves, side by side, and run your finger along one of the halves, feeling its moisture. Lick your finger. Now pick up one of the halves and bite or suck it. Can you feel its acidic juices on your tongue? Is there anyone who is not salivating yet? You did this simply through your thoughts, which control the state of your mind, which, in turn, affects your body's responses, in this case providing the saliva that would be required in your mouth to eat a lemon. And it was done through your thoughts alone! Imagine how this powerful and natural way of thinking can be used to achieve your goals, such as ideal weight, overall health and physical well-being.

Success starts with believing in yourself

Harnessing the power of your mind means maintainable, sustainable changes in your life, forever!

It's well documented that successful people have incredible self-belief and confidence in their ability. Henry Ford once said, 'Whether you think you will succeed or not, you are right.' And as you think about this, you will begin to see the truth in this simple statement. If you think you can, you can. And if you think you can't, you can't. The difference is nothing has meaning until you give it meaning. As a slimmer, knowing that you can and will achieve your healthy, happy weight, and stay there, is probably the most powerful tool.

Think slim to become slim

Basically, there are only two steps to making a change. First, change your perception so that the meaning you put to something makes you feel different. Second, change your behaviour, which comes out of your new thinking. This means that you behave differently and this gets you new results. In other words, you are thinking yourself slim! As you think it, so you become it, by behaving in a way and making the choices that support your thoughts. If you begin to think of yourself as a fit, energetic and healthy all-rounder, you are far more likely to make behavioural choices, including what you eat and drink, in accordance with this core belief. Then you're more likely to choose the juicy apple over the gooey chocolate bun because it fits in with your view of yourself as a healthy person. If you just attempt to change your eating habits without changing your thinking, you are likely to fall at the first hurdle.

Working with changes that alter the way you see yourself will bring about lasting, consistent behaviour – as opposed to short-term quick fixes! Through practice and repetition, you can condition your new thinking and actions to become automatic. Before you know it, making healthy lifestyle and food choices becomes second nature. Somebody once said, 'Here's how to get what you want – do whatever it takes!' So, if you want to stop biting your nails, stop putting your fingers in your mouth!

Managing your weight is not just about knowing what goes on your plate. New skills, such as using your mind to work with you, developing amazing will-power, the language you use, what you say to yourself, and understanding hunger, are all keys to successful weight control. We'll train you to use your mind to flick the switch that enables you to opt for the healthier choice, because *you* want to and because *you* know it will bring *you* the extraordinary results you want. And we give you the knowledge to help you decide which foods to reach for in simple, practical, no-nonsense language. So it's as easy as 1-2-3: Start-it, Lose-it and Keep-it … forever.

The story of the moth

Doing what you always do and expecting a different set of results would come close to a definition of insanity – a fried egg short of a full English! The story of the moth illustrates the challenge of achieving what you set out to achieve. The moth is attracted to the light indoors and flies towards it, but keeps banging against the window pane. Unless it changes its approach, the result remains the same. So how does this relate to making the right food choices? Put simply, if you want to achieve your goal of attaining your happy weight, you'll need to examine your approach and make conscious decisions to change the foods you select.

- Decide what it is that you really want.
- Do something about it – take appropriate action.
- Notice what's working and what's not working and act accordingly.
- Keep changing your approach (unlike the moth), until you get what you set out to achieve.
- Know that with this positive mental attitude, you can only succeed.

Dieting makes you fat!

What are your immediate thoughts when you hear the word diet? For many, it conjures up food deprivation, hard work, avoiding pleasurable sensations and

As soon as you have to avoid a food, you want it even more! Use your new thinking to reach the goals you want.

more. What happens when you say to yourself that you shouldn't eat a certain food? That food becomes even more desirable, let's face it. Many diets offer you weight loss if you avoid this and that food, but the more you're told to avoid it, the more you want it! Think back to when this might have been true for you. It's no wonder that you inadvertently sabotage the very goal that you set out to achieve by devouring the very food you're 'not supposed' to have. Think about it. If you are programming your brain into thinking that a diet means food deprivation, your mind is likely to rebel against any diet before it's begun! So part of the trick here is to make the weight-loss goal as enjoyable, pleasurable and as much fun as possible.

Link pleasure to dieting and you'll be surprised how much easier it is to reach your happy weight in a safe and sustainable way. In your mind, connect this change with your choice of low-GI foods and a change in lifestyle, so that eating healthily becomes a natural, everyday part of your life. So, how do you transform pain into pleasure? Try our booster tips.

Booster tips

- Make a list of the long-term benefits that your new lifestyle will give you. For example, a general feeling of being well, an increase in self-confidence, looking and feeling great about yourself, a lowering of blood cholesterol and an increase in energy levels.

- Indulge and challenge your creative side – give it another airing! Think about the healthy, tasty foods that do it for you. Yes, that's right, you can have your cake and eat it too. Remember to choose foods that support you in reaching your goal, by focusing on the new you. Use our menu tips to put your own tailor-made eating plans together. Share them with family and friends. What you think about influences your behaviour, so thinking and choosing more foods from the low- and medium-points section will naturally help you to attain that result earlier on.

- Take a moment to consider what's really important. Ask yourself this question: 'Is the choice that I am making right here and now taking me closer to achieving what's truly important to me?' Whether it's the bar of chocolate, or the apple, that extra glass of something, or that éclair, choose wisely, knowing that different choices carry different consequences. Today's choices determine what happens tomorrow.

- You can support your thinking by finding a photo of how you would like to look, one that expresses the 'new' you. By looking at it when you feel like straying, it will remind you of what you can achieve.

Don't think about kangaroos!

You will now find that you cannot stop yourself from thinking about kangaroos! Your mind finds it hard to recognise a negative command and so deletes it, acting upon the last instruction that it was given, in this case: think about kangaroos. This helps explain why if you tell yourself, or someone else, not to worry, the worry expands. Or, as is common with parents, telling a child not to spill its drink increases the chances of the drink being spilt. Thinking about what you really do want, as opposed to your 'don't wants', will increase your chances of getting it. In this case, 'Hold the cup tightly!'

Top sports people have become skilled in this way of thinking. They know that if they think of serving the ball into the net, or kicking the ball at the goalpost, then chances are that's exactly where it will end up. Instead, they think of the result as a done deal. They see the result exactly as they wish it to be, hearing the cheers from their fans and feeling the elation of the achievement. This same principle applies to your health and food plan – and any other aspect of your life.

Dad's army

In his book *The Naked Leader*, David Taylor tells the following story. A soldier practised golf seven days a week, for several hours a day, and never missed a shot. The odd thing was, he was a prisoner of war at this time, cooped away in a cell that was barely big enough to swing a cat. After he had been captured he had realised that his sanity depended upon keeping his mind exercised, and so he chose his most loved sport, golf. Every day, he played a full 18 imaginary holes. Nothing was left to chance. Every tiny detail was lived and relived: the uniqueness of the course itself, what he wore, the sounds around him – from the birds' chorus, to general conversations – and the different smells that each changing season brought with it. He felt the club firmly in his hands, and practised each swing until it was spot on. As he did so, he watched every ball bounce and roll to its imagined place. Every step that he carried out in his mind's eye took up the same amount of time as if it were for real.

Fortunately, he survived to tell the tale and went on to discover that he had knocked many, many strokes off his handicap, without having set foot on a golf course in several years.

Your energy flows to whatever you focus your attention on. Your mind is wonderfully programmed to devote more to what it is that

Energy flows to whatever it is that you focus on

you are thinking about. So if you are thinking about not wanting to put on weight, extra weight is exactly what you'll get. Inadvertently, by thinking about your 'don't wants' you are programming yourself to get more of the same. It's like being in a dirty wash cycle, going round and round! The great news is that there is a way out. With a little practice (it's that magic word, again!), you can begin to achieve the results that you really want, by remaining mindful of how you are thinking. When you catch yourself thinking about all the things that you don't want, for example, 'I don't want to be overweight', ask yourself what it is that you *do* want, instead. This question is a critical turning point. For example say to yourself, 'I choose to be slim, energetic and confident.' What and how you think influences what you create, which becomes your reality.

It's a goal!

Having goals is what keeps us going. Yours may include reaching a happy weight, becoming healthier, fitter and going about your business with great energy. Goals remind you that you're still alive. Goals and outcomes provide us with momentum, anticipation, direction and flow. How often do you hear of great achievers and other successful people who, having retired, lose their reason for living? It happens and it's only too common. Whatever your goal, be clear about what it is and develop a real sense of the burning desire behind it.

There are many magnificent stories about people accomplishing what many of us would think of as being almost impossible. They weren't necessarily the most intelligent, strongest or bravest people. They just had a hugely compelling desire to get somewhere and that was enough! It's this kind of thinking that, when applied to your weight-loss goals, will enable you to get there, too.

Your journey is as important as your destination

Some people procrastinate so much before choosing the 'right' goals and getting everything perfect that they are near to pushing up the daisies by the time they decide! Then it's too late. Now is all you have, it's the 'gift' of the moment. That's why it's called the 'present'.

Enjoying the journey is one of the all-important parts of the process. Who you become along the way, what you learn and what you experience are more important than arriving! What's the point if you didn't stop to admire the scenery, smell the flowers or appreciate the wind blowing across your face? The other common mistake is getting stuck on striving and so putting your life on hold. For example, the trap here is in thinking that once you lose weight, fit into that smaller dress size, find a new partner, get a more

> There is no failure – only feedback.

exciting job (and more!), life will be right! Hmmm. If you have the mental outlook to enjoy life now, then you'll more than likely have it in the future. If you don't, you won't! If all you've got guaranteed is what you have now, putting off being happy until some time in the future is as mad as a box of frogs!

Overwhelmed? Turn it around

If you feel like giving it all up, think about how great you'll feel when you get there, and simply start again. You're only human, and it's okay to have those 'off days'. Often in life, events occur that are outside of your control. Perhaps you've tried several approaches already and when you don't see immediate results, you give up. Nobody wants to give his or her all, only to be disappointed. You may even convince yourself that you've reached the point where nothing works and you're no longer even willing to try. This is described as 'learned helplessness'. The good news is that you can make changes in your life today by changing your *perceptions* and/or your *responses*.

You can start by focusing on what you can do *today* to make your life richer and, of course, this includes your health and well-being. You can consciously choose to be well, today. Whatever and whoever you have become, it is due to the accumulative thoughts that you have about yourself, about who you are. Your responses are a result of how you think of yourself, and your actions will be consistent with your thoughts. In other words, your identity governs your actions.

The story of the frog and the scorpion illustrates this delightfully!

The sting

Once upon a time, there stood a scorpion on the edge of the riverbank, trying to figure out a way to get across the water. His prayers were answered when he caught sight of a frog. 'Excuse me, Mr Frog,' he called. 'Please will you give me a ride on your back so I can get to the other side?' The frog looked startled and puzzled by the question. After a moment of deliberation, the frog told the scorpion that he couldn't possibly oblige as he was likely to get stung by the scorpion. On hearing this, the scorpion laughed out loud. 'Don't be silly, Mr Frog. If I were to sting you, I too would drown!' On reflection, albeit with some hesitation, the frog agreed and told the scorpion to hop on to his back. Just before reaching the

Think more and more about who or what you would choose to be like. Let your thoughts gravitate towards those choices.

other side, the scorpion stung the frog. As the drowning pair started to go down, the frog managed to ask why the scorpion had committed this act. The scorpion replied, 'Because that's what scorpions do, they sting!'

What has dieting done for you?

How many people do you know who, at some time in their lives, have been on a diet? And how many have kept the weight off? (Honest now …) The dieting industry in the UK is estimated to be worth over a billion pounds each year, and most of us are likely to have contributed to this in one way or another.

Has it made you slimmer? Has it improved your lifestyle? Has it made you able to resist the foods your diet asks you to avoid? People who diet tend to think about food a lot. They often step on the weighing scales at every opportunity. And they are sucked into the latest dieting trend. Could this be you?

If you continue to go for the latest quick fix, you'll continue to fall into the dieting trap. You'll be promised a huge weight loss in days or weeks, which is far more enticing than the slower weight loss the dietitians and medics will encourage. But, you know the facts – the steady, sensible weight loss is far healthier and works in the long term. And that's the GiP-effect.

Motivational power booster

Here's one of the best-kept secrets! Working with the following exercise could change your life. Try it daily, as many times as possible, if you're ready to make those sustainable and long-lasting changes. Be careful what you think about, as you are highly likely to get it!

Imagine yourself as the 'new' you that you most want to be. Study the picture in as much detail as you can, as if it had already happened. See yourself spending time with people who are supportive, fun and motivational. Like laughter, it's infectious! Visualise yourself being able to fit into your favourite jeans, being able to run after your kids (and catch them!), and doing things that previously you wouldn't have had the confidence to do.

Hear the comments others are making to you, now that you've achieved your goal. Hear their congratulations and other encouraging words. Say and repeat positive things to yourself, congratulating yourself on your achievements so far. What you say to yourself is key.

Feel the 'positivity' of your success and how these feelings and emotions make you feel so great about yourself. Feel that enhanced sense of energy and inner confidence growing. Remember what this is doing for you and the difference that it is making to others close to you, too. Perhaps you are now enjoying new and varied interests with your family and loved ones.

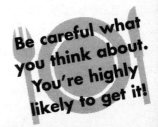

Be careful what you think about. You're highly likely to get it!

*Remember GiP Rule 6: Imagine the new you every day
– a past photograph will help.*

Helpful questions to ask yourself

- How will achieving this make me feel?
- What will be truly important to me about achieving this?
- How much more could I accomplish in other areas of my life?
- How could others benefit when I make these changes?
- How much happier will I feel?

You are the only one in control of your thoughts and actions. Do this exercise as many times in a day as you choose. Like working out at a gym, practice, repetition and conditioning is the key. You wouldn't expect to get that perfect body after one session in the gym. Similarly, changing your thinking to support your goals positively requires practice, too. You'll be amazed at the results, so enjoy it!

A family affair

The Ricchiuti family followed these principles, daily. The results within three months were amazing.

Dad opted for a healthy and balanced approach in

his food choices. He thoroughly looked forward to his daily workout sessions at the gym and his confidence grew considerably. He learnt to use a computer (previously a technophobe!) and began to communicate more openly with his lovely wife, which has enriched the quality of their relationship.

Mum lost the most weight and reached her happy weight effortlessly! As a result of this, her confidence and self-esteem grew considerably and this encouraged her to apply successfully for a new job that she so wanted. She was ecstatic! She'd landed her ideal job.

Their eight-year-old daughter developed a love affair with vegetables (she couldn't stand them before!), and now chooses them willingly, because she knows that they are good for her. Her teachers noticed that her concentration had improved 100 per cent, since she stopped having fizzy drinks.

Their son, 14 years old, is enjoying the improved relationship he has with his family and loves the increased fun activities that they now share. His skin has improved and he is noticeably enjoying eating a lot more fruit.

You may or may not wish to become an entrepreneurial leader, sail around the world single-handed or win a gold medal, but you will have at least one thing in common with those who do. Your goal will be so compelling and seductive that you cannot fail to achieve it! Before you go any further, commit to your very first step in achieving this goal and know exactly when you are going to take it. 'Excusitis' ends right here, right now!

New beginnings

Think about all the healthy, tasty foods that you want to eat, the foods that will support you in reaching your goal. You already know what you think influences your behaviour, so in your thinking, include the succulent cherries, the filling pasta in tomato sauce, the sweet potato and the grainy bread. Thinking about the new you also means you're focusing on what you want.

More steps to success

- If you do overindulge – enjoy it! This is not mad advice. It frees you from feelings of guilt and anger, which make many people abandon their diets. Afterwards, simply get back on track.

- Keep a food and mood diary (see page 332) to show what you ate, where, why, and how you felt at the time. You may find that you eat in response to stress or strong emotions.

- Become more active. Walk to work instead of driving, use the stairs instead of the lift, and take the dog for a walk.

- Try to make each meal an occasion to be enjoyed, sitting at the table, rather than stuffing down snacks at work or as you do the housework. Get into the habit of putting your fork down after every mouthful – it works wonders in helping you eat more slowly.

- Try to get your family and friends to support you. Tell them that you want to be slimmer and healthier.
- Brush your teeth after every meal or snack – it really helps you stop eating.
- Write down your goal. Make it specific. For example, 'I will weigh "x" on such and such a date.'
- Believe in yourself. Know that you can *only* succeed. Keep a daily reference diary to record every success, no matter how little or large.

And the mother of them all …

Picture your plate

You will remember from Chapter 1 that a great tip for helping you to choose wisely and to ensure that you have a balanced, slimming yet filling meal is to imagine your plate is split into quarters. Now, fill two

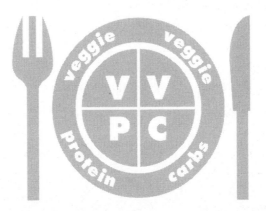

quarters with veg (such as crunchy broccoli and carrots), one with low-GI carbs (such as aromatic sweet potatoes), and one with protein (such as char-grilled meat or fish). Look at the picture on page 241 and take it with you in your mind whenever you sit down to a meal.

Using the 'really wants' philosophy, think now about how you can achieve this small goal, every time you have a meal.

See your plate perfectly proportioned and remind yourself of all the great results that this will bring you.

Summary

- The mind doesn't distinguish between what's real and what's imagined when you use all of your senses, so you feel that emotional intensity building.
- The mind doesn't easily recognise a negative command and acts on the last instruction that it receives.
- The mind is programmed to give you more of whatever it is that you are thinking about.

13

STRESS CITY

The wheelbarrow test

There is no stress out there, only people having stressful thoughts! If this is true, the first step is to consider *how* you are thinking about *what* you are thinking about. There is no stress out there, no depression and no fear. You cannot collect these up and put them in a wheelbarrow, can you? So where do those emotions come from? The answer is they come from the way you interpret circumstances or an event. For example, if you heard some bad news today, but the event happened a week ago, then it is not the event itself that causes you to feel bad. It is the meaning that you give it today, even though it took place sometime in the past!

Laugh a lot!

Row, row, row your boat gently down the stream.

Acquiring balance in all aspects of your life, and that includes maintaining a healthy diet, is to live your life in a state of well-being. Stress is a major contributor to comfort eating, bingeing and excessive drinking, and is responsible for a variety of illnesses. If you think about it, being ill at ease with yourself could be termed as being dis-eased. Becoming increasingly at ease with yourself and being happy, and liking yourself for who you are today, is another way to choose well-being. To help yourself and have a positive effect on those around you, there are a number of considerations that you may wish to think about as you explore how to become best friends with yourself. For example, when you're happy with who you are, you are less likely to punish yourself when you temporarily stray from your healthy lifestyle.

Penny for your thoughts

- Decide how you would recognise balance in your life. What would you see, hear and feel? Make a list.
- Decide on some specific and tangible tasks/actions that will achieve this – perhaps enlisting the support of others along the way.

- Notice what's working, or not working, regularly and make the necessary changes.
- Celebrate your efforts and results along the way!

Your body has an excellent built-in pharmacy where it produces, through your ideas, thoughts and responses, its very own powerful set of antibiotics, tranquillisers and other natural drugs. As you think, respond and experience, your body is simultaneously producing these chemicals. Tranquillity, for example, releases chemicals that help you relax (Valium without the side effects!). Similarly, exercise and laughter trigger the release of endorphins, which are powerful chemicals that are known to help you deal with stressful situations.

Your thoughts constantly reveal themselves through your body, your physiology. When you think and experience positiveness, joy, happiness and peace your appearance reflects this. You may, for example, smile or look at peace as your facial muscles relax and your breathing becomes deeper. If you were to think stressful thoughts, these would travel through your system to different parts of the body, making various muscles contract. This, too, can be seen on the outside, producing a different set of results.

Events don't create, they reveal

You may not always have control over all areas of your life, and that includes other people, but remember:

you always have control over how you interpret and respond to events. Mental flexibility is the key. Remove any mental barriers that are restricting the way you perceive the world. The following story illustrates the point.

A messy business!

Once upon a time there lived a father and his daughter. One day the daughter asked her father how it was that things got messed up so easily. The father asked what she meant. Pointing to her study, she explained that stuff was all over the place, messy and not perfect. It was, she said, only the previous evening that she had tidied up – but look at it now! The father, to try to understand, suggested that she showed him what it was like when things were in order. She duly did so by moving her things about until it resembled perfection in her eyes. The father then asked how it would be if he moved some bits and pieces a foot away from where she had placed them. She replied that it would once again be messy. Then he asked what it would be like if he left a book open and shifted another item to a different spot. Again, she responded that that too would be messy. The father concluded that it's not that things get messed up easily but that his daughter had more ways of interpreting things as being in a mess. He pointed out her pattern – she has only one way of viewing things as being perfect.

What's more important, being right or being happy?

'Let go' may be two small words, but put them together in the same sentence and they can be very powerful. There is an approach called 'the path of least resistance'. This suggests that learning to let go of always having to be right, of anger, frustration, bitterness, resentment, jealousy, and all the other negative feelings that prevent you from continuing on the path, will make an instant difference to your state of inner peace. The meaning that you put to what is happening in your life at any given time, and how you respond to it, is critical in shaping the experiences of your life. Remember that life is cyclical, like the four seasons. Everything comes, passes or changes and something else takes its place. Every time you let go of anything limiting, you are making space for something better.

Trick or treat?

Despite life's adversities, choosing a sense of well-being means looking at all the good things that already exist in your life. One person will look out of the window and notice the glorious scenery. Another might pay more attention to the dirty pane of glass. You can choose to have preferences in your life and still be grateful for what shows up!

Be prepared to look for the 'pay-off' in any situation or relationship. If you are miserable about all the things that you want but haven't got, think about all the things that you don't want and haven't got! There is a positive side to everything – the trick is to be open to seeing it. Be creative and think about all the ways you can truly enrich your life. This often starts with challenging your current way of perceiving things.

Perhaps you will now feel encouraged to think that every (so-called) adversity has the seeds of equal, or greater, benefit. Learn to trust what is happening in your life at any given moment. The richness and quality of your life experiences depends on the way you interpret events and circumstances. This is entirely within your control!

The following story illustrates this point.

A father and his son owned a farm. One day the only horse they owned ran away.

'What terrible bad luck,' the neighbours cried.

'Good luck, bad luck, who knows?' said the farmer.

Several weeks later the horse returned, bringing with him three wild mares.

'What excellent luck,' said the neighbours.

'Good luck, bad luck, who knows?' replied the farmer.

The son began to ride the wild horses and one day he was thrown and broke his leg.

'What bad luck,' said the neighbours.

'Good luck, bad luck, who knows?' replied the farmer in his enigmatic manner.

The following week the army came to the village to take all the young men to war. The farmer's son was still disabled with his injury and so was spared. Good luck, bad luck, who knows?

Life's challenges can also bring benefits – if you let them.

Choose P.E.A.C.E.

Perceive everything in your life as happening for a good reason and believe that nothing happens by chance.

Enjoy the present – a present is a gift! Live your life in the here and now.

Appreciate all that you have and be thankful for what you don't!

Contribute towards supporting others. Giving is receiving and it will make you feel great.

Eliminate conflict from your life by following the path of least resistance.

Believe it to see it

Consider this inspiring exercise to remind yourself of your hidden riches.

- Make a list of all the different aspects of the way you want to be. Decide how you will show these through your actions and in what you say. For example, if you choose to become more patient, think of an event that would normally get you hot under the collar, such as a traffic jam. Now, visualise yourself handling this with calmness. Put on your favourite music. Feel your face and body relaxing totally. Accept that there is nothing more powerful than controlling your emotions in a positive way. Leave the road rage to Mr Angry!

Ask yourself how you can use this knowledge to let go of your anxieties and stresses so that you can find peace. Put those concerns into a balloon and watch it float up and away until it disappears from view. Notice how much lighter you are already beginning to feel.

- Find a symbol to trigger this sense of release and remind you to let go of tension, which you can access at any time. Your symbol should be something attractive and meaningful to you like the balloon already mentioned. Alternatively it might be a piece of music, or an action such as taking a walk (walk off your worries) or a shower (wash away your stresses).

An attitude of gratitude

An attitude of gratitude ensures that you focus on what you really want. Remember: whatever you are thinking about, you're highly likely to get more of the same. Resist the tendency to focus on lack: what's missing, what's wrong and what you don't have. Instead, concentrate entirely on what is great and abundant in your life.

Develop an attitude of gratitude

Have you ever thought about buying a new car? Now as you look around on the roads, every other car seems to be the same model that you are after. Coincidence? Not so. It's simply that this is what you are focusing on. In order to attract good fortune, you need to feel fortunate. By doing so, you are more likely to be motivated towards achieving your new weight and a healthier you, and becoming a grand role model to others.

Life is right

Here are some special questions to ask yourself, daily:

- What am I happy about in my life today? What is it about this that makes me happy? How does that make me feel?
- What am I proud about in my life? What is it about that which makes me feel proud? How does that make me feel?
- What am I grateful for in my life? What is it about that which makes me grateful? How does that make me feel?
- Who do I love? Who loves me? How does that make me feel?

Every day, in every way, I feel amazing!

● What am I enjoying most in my life? What is it about that which I enjoy? How does that make me feel?

Draw on the present, or on the past, to help you actually feel the emotions. If you have difficulty with this, act as if it is true, by pretending!

Affirmations

An affirmation is an uplifting, motivational and positive thought, repeated as many times as you choose, daily. It's a fast track to the unconscious, the real driver of your thoughts. Try it. For example, say, 'I feel healthy, fit and energetic.' Affirmations are even more effective when you say them out loud or write them down. This ensures your mind really is on the affirmation itself, rather than thinking about your next snack! Repetition is very important. You may be changing a pattern that you've held on to for years but is now past its sell-by date!

A recipe for happiness

The greatest gift you can give another is to be responsible for your own happiness, as opposed to placing the burden on someone else's doorstep.

Taking responsibility, letting go and forgiving others is a way of choosing to live in the present, rather than remaining stuck in the past. Forgiving yourself can be challenging too. You might think that you don't deserve to be happy, healthy, slim, or have high self-esteem. That outlook can lead to over-eating, excess drinking, or failed relationships. You have suffered enough. You are your own worst critic. Choose to let it go. Make up your mind to move on, and act on this decision. Maintaining a healthy mind and body *is* worth the time, cost and effort. Blame and guilt keep you where you are, avoiding the real issue. So, make the change. Think positive!

You cannot be serious!

Laughter is the best medicine, it's official! When you are having fun, you are far more uplifted, determined and motivated towards your goal, the new you. Laughter produces a healthy dose of endorphins, which give you feelings of happiness and well-being and lessen the effect of stress hormones.

Take laughter seriously! Children can be your greatest teachers and you can rediscover life through a child-like state. Their intuitive hunger for joy and fun keeps them naturally balanced and healthy. As you grow up, the spontaneity can get knocked out of you. Choosing to apply humour, playfulness and a sense of joy to everyday life, taking yourself and life less seriously, encourages all kinds of wonderful things that benefit your body and mind.

Now take a moment to:
See the new you with a spirit of joy and lightness surrounding you.
Hear the laughter and the giggles coming from within you and the people around you and **feel** the surge of lightness and joy, in abundance.

ZZZzzz

Having a restful, good night's sleep contributes to your overall sense of well-being and enhances your ability to perform well, as you go about your business and daily life. You are far more likely to remain energised and alert throughout the day and therefore more able to cope with life's little challenges!

Here are some tips that can help you develop a good sleep pattern.

- Go to bed when you feel sleepy. You can't force your mind into sleep.
- Your bed is your haven. Associate your bed with calming the mind – your quiet time.
- If you're still lying awake after 30 minutes or so, get up and do something that will make you feel sleepy, such as reading a boring book, or writing a letter.

● Eat a light meal in the evening and avoid caffeine and alcohol too close to bedtime.

Clearing your mind

Let go of your day's worries and frustrations before you go to bed. In your mind, parcel them up and tie them on to the end of a very large, brightly coloured kite. Holding on to the kite's string, ask your subconscious (it likes to be helpful) to find solutions while you enjoy a peaceful night's sleep. Now fly the kite. See it rising and soaring higher and higher, without a care in the world, dancing up in the sky with an enviable sense of freedom. Now release the kite and trust that your request will be actioned.

Remember, for every worry there is a solution. If you are worrying about being overweight, the solution is to be slim, trim and bouncing around with vitality and energy. Using that principle of positive thinking, vividly imagine what you would look like. Think of the compliments that others would pay you. Really allow yourself to feel great as you experience what it is like to have achieved this outcome. As you do so, think of at least one small step that you can take the very next day, with certainty, that will help you get nearer to your goal.

Simplify your life

Simplify, simplify, simplify your life!

Clearing the clutter in your life can reduce stress by enhancing the flow of energy. Your home and working space is a reflection of you. So, while you are putting your house in order (literally!), you are also dealing with your internal clutter. The two go hand in hand. By removing any unwanted obstacles, you will promote harmony in other aspects of your life, making room for new and rich experiences to enter.

Testing for clutter

Think about the various objects, items of clothing and other bits and bobs that fill your home. Now ask yourself the following about each item:

- Does it make me feel good when I see it?
- How useful is it to me, *now*?
- Do I really appreciate it or love it?

If not, bin it and make room for something else!

Let go of your limitations and create space for something better.

My cup overfloweth

A student, who had dedicated his life to the quest for spirituality and the meaning of life, heard that the Master of all spiritual beings could be found in a distant place. The student set off on his mission to find this one, supreme Master. This being would finally give him the answer to his life's mission. He trekked the rocky paths, climbed mountains as high as they were wide, and travelled the seven seas, until he arrived at his destination. Cutting his way through the rain forest, he came across an unimpressive wooden hut, in the middle of nowhere. Here he found his guru. Bowing gracefully and barely able to make eye contact, he asked the burning question that had brought him. The Master smiled knowingly and asked him if he would share in a cup of tea. The student, hiding his puzzlement and impatience, nodded politely. The Master started pouring and continued pouring and pouring and pouring until the student exclaimed, 'Master, my cup overfloweth!' 'Yes,' said the guru. 'You have crammed so much in that you haven't room for anything new or fresh to enter into your life.' The student got it! Now he, too, was ready to become a Master.

Sorted!

- Surround yourself with things that bring you happiness and promote a feel-good flow of energy.

- Clutter creates stress and confusion, rather than the peace of mind that comes from knowing where things are. Have a clear-out.
- Tackle problems in your home and in your life. Closure can be liberating, promoting a positive flow of harmony and energy.

Junk out your home, junk out your body

Perhaps there is a correlation here. Once you've cleared the junk out of your physical space, it's easier to stop putting it in your body! The extra fat that you are carrying acts as a protective cushion. Similarly the junk you have accumulated in your home could be there to cushion you against the emotional turmoil of life. Letting go of the junk allows you to let go of the weight. Whatever you have created in your life up to now is there for a reason and has served a purpose. Re-evaluate the situation and start over. New broom, clean sweep. Open up to the freshness of new beginnings.

Three tips for a mental clear-out

- Park your criticism, judgement and any gossip! When you criticise others you are simply defining something about yourself that you don't accept and projecting it on to someone else! What you think of me is none of my business! As for gossip, well, this is a complete waste of time. Live and let live. It's part of accepting life and its flow.

● Deal with loose ends. For example, if you get a letter, action it, file it, or bin it – whatever is appropriate. Do it today and don't put it off until tomorrow! This applies to other loose ends that may be depleting your valuable energy, such as returning something you borrowed or repaying a debt, writing a letter, or making a phone call.

● Avoid diary envy! Do you define success by how much 'busyness' you have scheduled in your diary, compared with everyone else? You have a choice to go the other way and make 'you' time a priority. The rest can be made to fit in around this. If you do virtually nothing other than work and take care of others, tiredness and lack of well-being will soon become apparent. By taking care of you, you'll be that much more able to look after others, be it your partner, family, friends or colleagues. Your soul needs nourishment, too: it's what makes you blossom.

Three tips for an emotional clear-out

● Let go of any grievances. Forgive and forget and make the decision to get on with your life. Grievances keep you stuck in the past and it costs valuable energy hanging on to them. They eat

Surround yourself with joyful people.

away at you over time. Let go and get on with your precious life and open up to all the potential joy that is waiting to come in.

● Soul mate? Have the courage to follow your gut feelings. When you've given your relationship every chance of success, know in your heart when it's time to release both of you. Perhaps your journey is only meant to be shared with that person for part of the way?

● Friends? If you were to be truly honest now, how many friends would you rather let go of? And, as everyone you know has a list, whose lists are you on? Who are the negative people who are draining your energy? Instead, mix with wonderful, generously inspiring people who will fill your life with joy and freshness. Remember, your friends are an expression of you.

Tips for experiencing inner calm

● Laugh at your misfortunes. Everything happens for a reason. Trust that this is so.

● Encourage natural spontaneity in yourself, your kids and others. Laugh as much as possible. Watch funny films, hang out with happy people and let the children in your life become your role models and your teachers!

● Avoid the people and situations that bring about stressful thoughts.

● Identify whatever is causing you to become stressed and make a list of the changes you need to make. For example, is the problem to do with your eating habits, self-esteem, motivation or health? Is it the state of your relationships, your finances or your career – what needs to change?

● Close your eyes for a few minutes and go to a place in your mind's eye that you love and that makes you feel good. Choose somewhere that you associate with happy, calm and relaxing memories. Now see yourself as if you are there again. Look around you, notice the colours and as much detail as you can. Be aware of sounds and smells. Notice and relish the wonderful emotions that this evokes in you as you feel your whole body relaxing. Stay here for a few minutes. It's a great way of bringing balance back into your busy day.

● Treat yourself to a massage, including your feet. This will boost your circulation and reduce muscle tension.

● Take up a hobby or interest that you've always wanted to do. Doing what you love and loving what you do should apply to every area of your life.

● Bring happy thoughts into all that you do, daily. Happiness isn't a destination – it's a way to travel.

- Remember that the stress you are feeling at the moment will pass. Life is cyclical, like the natural laws of nature, the ebb and flow of the tide and the passing of the four seasons. Know that stress too shall pass.
- Finally, 50 per cent of what you worry about you can do something about, and 50 per cent of what you worry about you can't do anything about. Now you have nothing to worry about.

Boosting your immunity

Try this simple and relaxing visualisation to optimise your immune system.

- Close your eyes, relax and take slow, deep breaths.
- Feel a sense of health, vitality and energy flowing throughout your body.
- Imagine allowing a ray of bright, white light to enter through the crown of your head and flow throughout your body.
- Now direct this glowing light to the specific regions in the body where you are suffering pain or injury and see that light spreading and doing its job.
- Feel the intensity of this experience and then increase that feeling, double it and notice how great you are beginning to feel.
- Bask in the warmth of the flow of this light and then allow it out through the soles of your feet.

- Carry this great state with you as you go about your everyday life, knowing that it has made a difference.
- Find a few minutes (that's all it takes) to do this daily.

On the piste!

Annie had first-hand experience of this visualisation exercise with results that were so remarkable she could hardly believe it herself! In her case, she applied this technique when she fell and badly injured her knee in a skiing accident. This visualisation, directed towards her specific injury, enabled her to walk painlessly within a few minutes, and within a day she was back on the slopes enjoying and embracing her new-found power.

Annie's case is a real-life example of how, with practice, your thoughts and visualisations can influence your health. Such is the power of your mind in boosting a sense of well-being throughout your body.

Summary
- Thinking tranquil thoughts releases chemicals in your body that help you relax.
- You have control over the way you perceive your life.
- Look for the good things that already exist in your life.

14

QUESTIONS & ANSWERS

Q *I've tried many diet books – how do I really know this is not just another fad (here today, gone tomorrow) diet on the market?*

A When you buy a car, do you get a feel for the honesty of the dealer? Well, when you buy a diet book, gauge the credentials of the authors. Trust only those who are professionals and who have sound experience and backing. Registered dietitians are governed by a strict code of conduct, so if the author (like here) is a registered dietitian, that's a stamp of quality. Look for the letters RD after the name.

Q *How long before I can expect to see/feel/hear results?*
A The effects will be almost immediate as long as you've stuck to your Gi Point Diet. Each day counts as part of the accumulative effect and by the end of the week we would expect you to have lost up to 1 kg (2 lb), which is the safe and sustainable amount that we encourage.

Q *Can I still go out to eat? If so, what can I order at an Indian/Chinese/Italian/French restaurant?*
A The beauty of GiP is that you can continue to enjoy eating out, one of the little pleasures of life. We have dedicated a whole chapter to eating out (page 111), which covers all of the above.

Q *What if friends ask me to dinner? Do I warn them in advance what I can/can't eat? If I stop the diet when I'm, for example, on holiday, will all my good work be undone?*
A Nothing is out of bounds, just be mindful of your daily allowance of points. For the same reason, being on holiday means that you can continue to eat well by choosing your foods in line with the GiP Diet. Take your Gi Point Diet book with you and use the tables, smart shopping and menu planning (Hasty and Tasty) chapters to ensure healthy, tasty choices. And if you lapse a little, that's okay – you're on holiday.

Q *Do I have to buy lots of expensive foodstuffs?*
A No. The fab thing about how this works is that you

can buy what is within your budget. Our advice is to buy the best food you can, that suits your pocket. Check out the Smart Shopping chapter.

Q *Do I have to keep track of points and calories?*

A Yes and no – you keep track of the points, we take care of the calories. It's easy because we've done all the complicated maths for you. All you do is tot up your GiP allowance for the day. Simple as 1-2-3!

Q *Can kids and older people safely follow this diet?*

A Yes, with the guidance of a registered dietitian so that the number of points is right for the age group.

Q *How safe is this diet in terms of cholesterol?*

A The foods recommended in the GiP system are designed to be lower in fat, especially the saturated fat that has a strong influence on your blood cholesterol. Foods high in soluble fibre (such as beans, lentils and oats) have been shown to lower blood cholesterol. These are also low-GI foods. Always seek the advice of your GP if you have a medical condition.

Q *Will I feel tired when I first start the diet?*

A You might find that you've never felt better! This isn't a fad diet, which restricts your calories to very low levels. Use the guidelines to achieve balance and variety, keep to the number of points and see how you go. If you are losing weight too quickly, increase your points – see

Chapter 3. Obviously, if you do feel tired or unwell, check with your GP.

Q *How does it differ from other diets?*
A Each diet has its own guidelines and principles. A diet plan which incorporates a range of healthy foods from all the main food groups (carbs, proteins, fruit and veg, and dairy foods) plus an exercise recommendation is a good sign. The Gi Point Diet is based on good principles – and qualified nutritionists and dietitians use GI routinely.

Q *What sort of real changes will I have to make in my life for this to work?*
A The real change is making up your mind to make the change and following through on it by taking appropriate action. We have built in tried and tested highly motivational tools, coupled with some 'mental gymnastics' to make it all effortless for you.

Q *Will this be detrimental to my body/system over the long term?*
A The opposite is true. It will enhance your health and well-being through eating in a balanced and healthy way. Just make sure you vary the foods you choose and keep to the GiP rules.

Q *If this is so good, why has no one else come up with the idea before?*

A GI has been around for a long time. It just took us enormous time and effort to show that, once put into user-friendly, simplified tables, it is a practical system that can be used successfully by both men and women.

Q *Will this be an expensive diet to maintain?*
A No. Its flexibility allows for whatever you already put aside for your weekly food shop. Shopping on the internet may mean you spend less as you're not so tempted by the special offers.

Q *How do I maintain my weight once I have lost the pounds?*
A Good question! This is a lifestyle change, for the better. You simply up the number of points in your allowance and gauge your weight regularly. See Chapter 3 for more details.

Q *How easy is the diet to do?*
A It's easy as pie! We've done all the hard work for you. Simply read what the diet's about (page 3), follow our shopping tips (Chapter 4) and menu planning advice (Chapter 5). Look up the tables for the foods you want and the rest just falls into place. If you think it'll be easy, it will, and if you don't, it won't!

Q *Will I need to take supplements/nutrients alongside the diet?*
A The diet is designed to include a range of foods, which will help you achieve all-round good nutrition.

However, you might want to take a supplement as a safety net, in case you're not very good at eating a varied diet. Only choose a supplement that offers no more than 100 per cent of the RDA (Recommended Daily Allowance) of vitamins and minerals (see Chapter 9).

Q *Can you guarantee that I will lose weight on this diet?*
A We can't, but *you* can by following the GiP rules on food choices and physical activity.

Q *What sort of research is there on GI?*
A The research on GI is extensive, which is why we've built in a separate section at the back of the book for those interested in the science behind it all. And that is only a fraction of the studies that are out there.

Q *How long will it take me to get down to my ideal weight?*
A We would recommend that you aim for no more than 0.5–1 kg (1–2 lb) per week.

Q *Will I lose weight straight away?*
A We would expect you to lose at least 1 kg (2 lb) in weight by the end of your first week, provided you have followed our recommendations.

Q *I have been overweight for the last 20 years and have been on many boom and bust diets. How do I know this one is different and won't affect my health?*

A Many diet books do not offer the uniqueness of our powerful motivational boosters. Knowledge is not enough unless it is supported by a positive approach and mental attitude, which make the changes in your lifestyle sustainable. Couple this with a diet plan compiled by expert dietitians and you're well on your way to a healthier new you. The dietary guidelines in Chapter 9, Eating for Complete Health, are based on dietary recommendations from the Food Standards Agency and the British Dietetic Association. Balancing your carbs and proteins within a low-saturated-fat diet is integral to the Gi Point approach. If you are at all concerned about starting the diet, it is always best to seek the advice of your doctor.

Q *How do I prevent myself eating when I'm not really hungry?*
A The good news about GiP is that since you're eating three meals and three snacks daily you don't feel hungry! And if you do, there are plenty of GiP-free goodies to keep you going. Remember too that distraction works effectively. Take your mind off it by doing something else that you enjoy which is healthy, such as exercise, reading or making a phone call. There are many great tips throughout the book.

Q *I am a comfort eater. What can I do to control this?*
A If it's comfort that you are in need of, find another way of getting this pleasure in a more functional way. Try a bubble bath, music, a game of pool or meditation.

Q *I eat when I'm bored. What tips can you offer?*

A It is common to eat when you have a need that is unmet and boredom is one of them. Find other ways to relieve the boredom. There are many suggestions in the book. And if you want to eat, just choose a GiP-free snack (see page 103).

Q *I'm overwhelmed by the changes that I'd need to make to my whole lifestyle to make this work. Is there a quick and easy way?*

A This diet is designed, along with our tips on exercise, to fit in effortlessly with your lifestyle. By making bite-size changes daily, you'll accomplish your goal easily.

Q *Sometimes I feel that my body is 'stuck' and sluggish. What practical tips are there?*

A Physical activity works wonders for the mind and the body, which are linked. Turn to page 203 for tips. It's fab for beating the blues, too.

Q *I'm not sure that I can handle the expectations that I have about myself when I'm slim. What do you suggest?*

A You won't know until you've tried. Be that person today, ahead of time. See yourself as the new you and become him/her, as if you've **already** achieved your goal. Now think about what these expectations are and how the new, more confident, energetic you would handle these. More about this in Chapter 12.

Q *How do I get round not offending my hosts, partner, family and so on … by leaving food on the plate when I'm full?*

A Do what you can to make sure that you get served smaller portions, or serve yourself. If you want to have seconds that's great, provided, of course, that it's within your daily point allowance!

Q *How do I stay motivated?*

A Chapter 12 is dedicated to motivation and booster tips. Some of them are still the best-kept secrets, until now!

Q *How can I raise my level of motivation when it's down?*

A Think about what achieving your goals will do for you and how your life will be different. Refer to Chapter 12 on motivation and the tips throughout the book.

Q *Most of my mates eat and drink excessively when we're out. How do I resist the temptations?*

A Be focused on your outcome, not theirs! There's a satisfaction in knowing that you'll be the one waking up without that distended tum or blinding headache, not to mention having a mouth that tastes like a parrot's cage!

Q *I feel that I'm so overweight, how do I kick-start my motivation?*

A Take each day as it comes and do whatever it takes in even the smallest of ways to achieve small goals along the way. Keep an old picture of yourself somewhere prominent to remind you of what the new you will look like.

Q *I feel that my weight is linked with other stuff that is going on in my life. How do I go about sorting this out?*

A Food fills a physical hole, not an emotional need. Understanding what the other stuff is, that clutters your life, is the place to start. Take one issue at a time to simplify and declutter your life. Read Chapter 13 on stress for some of the best guidance, ever!

Q *I'm expecting myself and my life to be very different when I'm the 'right' size. How realistic is this?*

A The trick here is to enjoy your life as it is in the now. Visualising how you want it to be in the future will increase the likelihood, so make it as ideal as you would wish for.

Q *I've a suspicion that deep down something stops me from wanting to reduce my size. Can you help?*

A There is a pay-off in keeping things as they are. If there wasn't, you would have made the change already. Work out what it is that stops you and, with our guidance, build it into your outcome, in a healthy way.

Q *When I am infatuated or fall in love, my appetite is automatically suppressed. How do I avoid ballooning later on in the relationship?*

A Love and infatuation can act as natural appetite suppressants. You're full up with pleasurable feelings, so you tend to eat less. Ballooning later suggests that you are then trying to fill emotional needs with food, which doesn't work. Understand what the emotional needs are, talk these through with your partner, and move on.

Q *My partner cooks wonderful meals and gets irritable about my new eating regime. Any tips around dealing with this?*

A Open communication is the thing. Get him/her on your side, supporting you, and who knows? They may join in too.

Q *I don't eat when I'm stressed and so tend to lose weight, which is great. However, remaining in this state isn't a healthy way to do it. How can I make it easy at other times?*

A Set about de-stressing your life, so that you encourage a healthy flow of energy in and around you. Find functional ways to motivate yourself. There are loads in the book.

Q *How do I know this is really, really going to work and what else have I got to do besides follow the diet?*

A If you follow the simplicity of the points system, it will work. The Glycaemic Index is backed by a great deal of scientific research. Please refer to the various credible opinions and the additional appendices of science at the back of the book. The GiP Diet, in conjunction with regular activity, is a cracking combination for success.

Q *Why do low-GI foods keep us full for longer?*
A If you like your facts, you may want to know that when the blood-glucose level rises, the body responds by releasing a hormone, insulin, from the pancreas. This is called the insulin response. Insulin transports the glucose from the blood to muscle and fat stores for later use as energy. This then reduces the level of glucose in the blood. The faster a food raises blood-glucose levels, the greater the insulin response, resulting in a rapid fall in blood glucose. This is associated with hunger. So, the more foods you eat that cause a slow rise in blood glucose, the less hungry you are likely to feel.

Glucose also comes from other foods, but mainly from the starchy and sugary foods you eat. With new scientific evidence, we now know that not all carbohydrate foods have the same effect on blood glucose. The amount and type of fat, the type of fibre and even the way food is cooked or processed is more important.

Q *What affects GI?*
A Lots of things. Here are some of them. The structure and texture of the carbohydrate affects its GI. Pasta and durum wheat have a low GI. Wholegrains

and other high-fibre foods act as a physical barrier that slows down the absorption of carbohydrate. This is not true for 'wholemeal', however, for even though the whole of the grain is included, it has been ground up instead of being left whole. Stoneground wholemeal, which has slightly coarser grains, is better than a standard wholemeal. So, some mixed-grain breads that include whole grains have a lower GI than either wholemeal or white breads.

The GI of a food is affected by:

- The physical form of a food, such as the fibrous coat around beans, food being left whole, rather than being mashed.
- Finely milled flours have a faster rate of digestion. So, fine-ground flour made into bread (such as wholemeal) has a higher GI than granary.
- Soluble fibre has a low GI.
- Sugar is quickly digested, especially when it is in liquid form. So, sugary drinks, and foods with a high sugar/low fibre content, tend to have a high GI. It's difficult to generalise, since foods react in different ways, depending on the other foods you eat with them. So, combining a sugary drink with a meal of jacket potato and baked beans will have a different GI from having the drink on its own.
- Fat slows down the rate of digestion, which explains why foods with a high fat content may have a low GI.

Our meal combos in the tables and meal swaps have been devised using a special formula to calculate the GI of that mixed meal, so you get the benefit of an overall lower GiP value.

Q *What actually happens in my body?*

A 'Whole foods', such as whole grains, and foods high in 'soluble fibre', such as soya beans, take longer to be broken down by the body and thus cause a slower rise in blood glucose. If you think how easy it is to digest puréed pea soup – which is already in small particles (and quite sloppy, though delicious!), clearly the body doesn't need to spend much time mashing this up before the soup is digested and ready to go into the bloodstream as glucose. Now, imagine how much longer it would take for you to digest whole peas.

The body needs to break down the skin before it even reaches the pulp of the peas. Then it needs to break that pulp down into a form that is small enough to enter the bloodstream. So, whole peas will make the blood glucose rise much more slowly than the puréed soup. This is the case with most foods – for example, hummus compared with a whole chick pea casserole, mashed potatoes compared with a boiled potato, and wholemeal bread compared with seeded bread.

PART THREE

THE GI POINT TABLE

HOW TO USE THE Gi POINT TABLE

Here is your list of everyday foods along with their points value. The tables are laid out so you can find what you need quickly. There are two sets of tables.

In the first table, entries are arranged in ascending order of GiPs, and are split into the following groups:

- Meal carbs – choose one at each meal.
- Proteins – choose 2–3 portions each day.
- Vegetables.
- Fruits, desserts, snacks and drinks.
- Free flavourings.
- Fatty and sugary foods.
- Meal combos that save you points.
- Recipes that are low in points.
- Ready meals.

The second table is an alphabetical listing for quick reference – handy when you want to look up a particular food (see page 311) and you're in a rush.

(For ease of reference, 1 serving spoon = 3 tablespoons.)

The guidelines

1 The Gi Point Diet works because it helps to keep you full while you lose weight, and because it is based on a balanced range of healthy foods. In order to use the tables as they are intended, follow these simple guidelines:

- Eat three meals and three snacks every day.
- Choose fruit or other low-GiP foods for snacks.
- Keep to the instructions at the top of each page.
- Picture your plate in quarters and fill two quarters with vegetables (v, v), one quarter with protein (p) and one quarter with carbs (c) – remember: 'veggie, veggie, protein, carbs'.

2 Use the serving sizes to guide you – these are designed to fill you up and help you keep a watchful eye on nutrition. If you're cooking for more than one person, use what you need to cook, but make sure that what *you* eat is the portion size suggested.

3 Use GiP-free snacks *in addition* to low-GiP carbs, not instead of them.

4 We know that adding a low-GI food to a high one offers a reduction in the overall GI, which means your blood-glucose levels will be more stable, and you are less likely to feel hungry. Our healthy protein and carb meal combos have been calculated to take this extra benefit into account. And if you choose one of these combos, you enjoy a bonus reduction in points! If you were to simply add up the GiPs of the individual foods, you would notice that the GiPs are lower with the combos. That's because we've used a simple formula to take account of the benefit of combining foods: 'high + low = medium'. Always remember the golden rule of combining high-GiP carbs with low-GiP carbs.

5 Look out for lower-fat or reduced-sugar versions of the listed foods, as this will help you cut the calories.

6 For good long-term health, keep fatty and sugary foods to a minimum.

7 Some ready meals have been analysed by researchers for their GI, but this list is limited. To create low-GI culinary delights in a dash, cast your eyes over the recipe titles in the tables. The full recipes are given in Chapter 8.

8 If you are a whiz in the kitchen (or even if you're not), the points-free flavourings will give you a host of tempting ways to spice up plain foods – simply adding some chilli sauce to chick peas, or garlic to mushrooms, makes a tempting treat in seconds. If you find other flavourings that are virtually fat- and carb-free (check the label), go right ahead and add them to your list.

9 Remember the five-a-day fruit and veg mantra. The GiP-free vegetables and easy-peasy snack concoctions will help you achieve this effortlessly.

10 You will always have a daily allowance of 200 ml (⅓ pint) of semi-skimmed milk over and above your daily points total, so you can use this in drinks and in cooking without adding any extra points.

Food	Portion Size	GiPs	Special Comments

MEAL CARBS

(choose one at each meal)

BEANS AND LENTILS *(all beans and lentils count once a day as one of your five fruit and veg. These are also protein foods and if you choose them as your protein, then choose another carb)*

Food	Portion Size	GiPs	Special Comments
Chilli beans, canned	½ large can	1	
Haricot beans, dried, cooked	1 teacupful	1	
Lentils, red, split, dried, cooked	1 teacupful	1	
Blackeye beans, dried, cooked	1 teacupful	1.5	GI of some canned beans is not available
Butter beans, dried, cooked	1 teacupful	1.5	
Chick peas, whole, dried, cooked	1 teacupful	1.5	
Pigeon peas, whole, dried, cooked	1 teacupful	1.5	
Pinto beans, dried, cooked	1 teacupful	1.5	
Red kidney beans, dried, cooked	1 teacupful	1.5	you can use a combination of beans in smaller portions for the same points.
Soya beans, dried, cooked	1 teacupful	1.5	
Baked beans, canned in tomato sauce	small can	2	
Black gram, urad gram, dried, cooked	1 teacupful	2	
Mung beans, whole, dried, cooked	1 teacupful	2	
Red kidney beans, canned	½ large can	2	
Chick peas, canned	½ large can	2	great spiced up as a snack – add chilli sauce
Chick peas, split, dried, cooked	1 teacupful	2.5	
Broad beans, dried, cooked	1 teacupful	3.5	
Broad beans, canned	½ large can	4	
Broad beans, frozen, cooked	1 teacupful	4	

BREADS

Food	Portion Size	GiPs	Special Comments
Burgen oat bran, barley and honey bread	2 slices	2.5	
Burgen soya and linseed bread	2 slices	2.5	grains and seeds tend to lower the GI

Food	Portion Size	GiPs	Special Comments
Barley bread	2 slices	3	
Wheat tortillas	1 wrap	3	
Granary bread	2 slices	3.5	
Mixed-grain bread	2 slices	3.5	wholegrains are richer in B vitamins than refined grains
Pumpernickel bread	2 slices	3.5	
Barley and sunflower bread	2 slices	4.5	
Chapatis, made without fat	2 small chapatis	4.5	use coarse wholemeal flour
Rye bread	2 slices	4.5	
White bread, with added fibre	2 slices	4.5	
Hamburger buns	1 bun	5	
Pitta bread	1 pitta	5	wholemeal ones are higher in fibre
Chapatis, made with fat	2 small chapatis	5.5	
Hovis	2 slices	5.5	
White bread	2 slices	5.5	
Wholemeal bread	2 slices	5.5	opt for stoneground as it is more coarse and thus has a lower GI
Bagels, plain	1 bagel	6	a low-GiP carb (like sweetcorn) helps to reduce the GI of the meal
Melba toast, plain	2 toasts	7	
Taco shells, baked	1 shell	7	
Indian pooris	2 pooris	7.5	deep fried, so have on occasions only
Baguette	1 individual	9	a great food but a very high GI. Eat always with a low-GiP carb (like salad)

BREAKFAST CEREALS (see low-combo breakfasts, page 83)

Food	Portion Size	GiPs	Special Comments
All Bran and semi-skimmed milk	5 tablespoons+ 200 ml (⅓ pint)	2	try it with sliced banana
Porridge, made with water	8 tablespoons of made-up porridge as per pack instructions	3	

Food	Portion Size	GiPs	Special Comments
Porridge, made with milk and water	6 tablespoons of made-up porridge using 100 ml (¼ pint) milk and water as required	3.5	you could try skimmed milk, 200 ml (⅓ pint), instead. Use a little sweetener, honey or fructose if you like, add the GiPs
Muesli, reduced sugar and semi-skimmed milk	3 tablespoons+ 200 ml (⅓ pint)	4	
Special K and semi-skimmed milk	5 tablespoons+ 200 ml (⅓ pint)	4	
Bran Flakes and semi-skimmed milk	4 tablespoons+ 200 ml (⅓ pint)	4	
Muesli and semi-skimmed milk	3 tablespoons+ 200 ml (⅓ pint)	4	
Muesli, Swiss style, and semi-skimmed milk	3 tablespoons+ 200 ml (⅓ pint)	4	
Puffed Wheat and semi-skimmed milk	5 tablespoons+ 200 ml (⅓ pint)	4	
Instant hot oats made with semi-skimmed milk	follow pack instructions using 200 ml (⅓ pint) milk	4.5	a sachet at work could be a convenient breakfast
Shredded Wheat and semi-skimmed milk	2 biscuits+ 200 ml (⅓ pint)	4.5	
Weetabix and semi-skimmed milk	2 biscuits+ 200 ml (⅓ pint)	4.5	
Cornflakes and semi-skimmed milk	5 tablespoons+ 200 ml (⅓ pint)	4.5	
Nutrigrain and semi-skimmed milk	5 tablespoons+ 200 ml (⅓ pint)	4.5	
Grapenuts and semi-skimmed milk	5 tablespoons+ 200 ml (⅓ pint)	4.5	
Raisin Splitz and semi-skimmed milk	4 tablespoons+ 200 ml (⅓ pint)	4.5	
Sultana Bran and semi-skimmed milk	4 tablespoons+ 200 ml (⅓ pint)	4.5	
Rice Krispies and semi-skimmed milk	7 tablespoons+ 200 ml (⅓ pint)	5.5	

Food	Portion Size	GiPs	Special Comments

PASTA (most pasta is very low in GI. Use 50 g/2 oz raw per portion. Remember to add GiPs from sauces)

Food	Portion Size	GiPs	Special Comments
Fettucini, egg, cooked	5 tablespoons	1.5	
Spaghetti, white, cooked	5 tablespoons	1.5	
Spaghetti, wholemeal, cooked	5 tablespoons	1.5	
Macaroni, cooked	5 tablespoons	2	
Noodles, instant, cooked	5 tablespoons	2	
Linguini, thick, cooked	5 tablespoons	2.5	
Linguini, thin, cooked	5 tablespoons	2.5	
Noodles, rice, cooked	5 tablespoons	3	
Pasta, plain, cooked	5 tablespoons	3	

RICE AND GRAINS (keep rice grains whole rather than soft and mushy)

Food	Portion Size	GiPs	Special Comments
Rice, white, Bangladeshi, boiled	2 serving spoons	1.5	available from Asian grocers
Barley, pearl, cooked	1 teacupful	1.5	throw some into soups and stews
Bulgur, cooked	1 teacupful	2	
Rice, brown, boiled	2 serving spoons	2.5	
Rice, white, basmati, boiled	2 serving spoons	2.5	
Rice, white, precooked, microwaved	2 serving spoons	2.5	
Rice, white, easy cook, boiled	2 serving spoons	3	
Rice, white, instant, boiled	2 serving spoons	3.5	
Rice, white, polished, boiled	2 serving spoons	3.5	
Rice, white, risotto, boiled	2 serving spoons	3.5	
Couscous, cooked	1 teacupful	3.5	a nice change from rice
Semolina, cooked dry	1 teacupful	4.5	
Rice, white, glutinous (sticky), boiled	2 serving spoons	7	
Rice, white, jasmine, boiled	2 serving spoons	7.5	

SOUPS

Food	Portion Size	GiPs	Special Comments
Tomato soup, cream of, canned	1 soup bowl	1	
Instant noodle soup	1 soup bowl	2	
Lentil soup	1 soup bowl	2	

Food	Portion Size	GiPs	Special Comments

VEGETABLES – STARCHY *(these are part of meal carbs since they are high in starch. Other vegetables are not – you can find these under 'Vegetables')*

Food	Portion Size	GiPs	Special Comments
Plantain, boiled	1 plantain	1.5	available from West Indian food stores
Yam, baked	size of a medium potato	1.5	
Yam, boiled	size of a medium potato	1.5	
Yam, steamed	size of a medium potato	1.5	
Cassava, boiled	2 slices	2.5	available frozen in Asian food stores
Cassava, steamed	2 slices	2.5	
Breadfruit, canned, drained	2 slices	3	
Cassava, baked	2 slices	3	
New potatoes, boiled	4 new potatoes	3	keep skins on
New potatoes, canned, drained	4 new potatoes	3	
Old potatoes, boiled	3 egg-size potatoes	3	
Sweet potato, boiled	1 small potato	3	source of beta-carotene
Sweet potato, steamed or microwaved	1 small potato	3	
Breadfruit, boiled	2 slices	3.5	
Sweet potato, baked	1 small potato	3.5	
Matoki, boiled	1 matoki	4	available from Asian/West Indian grocers
Chips, straight cut, frozen, oven baked	2 serving spoons	5	choose 5% fat varieties
Cassava, gari	1 serving spoon	6	
Chips, French fries, fast food outlet	2 serving spoons	6	
Instant mashed potato made up with water	2 scoops	7	
Old potatoes, baked	1 medium potato	7	
Parsnip, boiled	2 tablespoons	7	serve with low GiP veggies
Parsnip, roast	2 tablespoons	7.5	

Food	Portion Size	GiPs	Special Comments

PROTEIN

(choose 2–3 portions a day)

BEANS AND LENTILS *(all beans and lentils count once a day as one of your five fruit and veg)*

Food	Portion Size	GiPs	Special Comments
Chilli beans, canned	½ large can	1	
Haricot beans, dried, cooked	1 teacupful	1	
Lentils, red, split, dried, cooked	1 teacupful	1	
Blackeye beans, dried, cooked	1 teacupful	1.5	
Butter beans, dried, cooked	1 teacupful	1.5	
Chick peas, whole, dried, cooked	1 teacupful	1.5	
Pigeon peas, whole, dried, cooked	1 teacupful	1.5	
Pinto beans, dried, cooked	1 teacupful	1.5	
Red kidney beans, dried, cooked	1 teacupful	1.5	you can use a combination of beans in smaller portions for the same GiPs
Soya beans, dried, cooked	1 teacupful	1.5	
Baked beans, canned in tomato sauce	small can	2	
Black gram, urad gram, dried, cooked	1 teacupful	2	
Mung beans, whole, dried, cooked	1 teacupful	2	
Red kidney beans, canned	½ large can	2	
Chick peas, canned	½ large can	2	great spiced up as a snack – add chilli sauce
Chick peas, split, dried, cooked	1 teacupful	2.5	
Broad beans, dried, cooked	1 teacupful	3.5	
Broad beans, canned	½ large can	4	great with red onion
Broad beans, frozen, cooked	1 teacupful	4	

EGGS *(max 5–6 per week, try omega-3 types)*

Food	Portion Size	GiPs	Special Comments
Eggs, boiled	2 eggs	1.5	
Eggs, poached	2 eggs	1.5	
Eggs, fried	2 eggs	3	
Eggs, scrambled, with milk and 1 tsp oil	2 eggs	3	
Omelette, plain, made with 1 tsp oil	2 eggs	3	

Food	Portion Size	GiPs	Special Comments
FISH (choose fish twice a week, one being oily fish which is rich in omega-3 fats)			
Cockles	6 cockles	1	
Cod, baked	1 fillet	1	
Cod, grilled	1 fillet	1	
Haddock, steamed or grilled	1 fillet	1	
Lemon sole, steamed or grilled	1 fillet	1	
Oysters	1 dozen oysters	1	shellfish are a good source of zinc, great for immune function
Plaice, steamed or grilled	1 fillet	1	
Prawns	1 small jar	1	choose fat-free dressing
Shrimps, canned in brine, drained	1 small pot	1	
Tuna, canned in brine, drained	small can	1	half the calories of canned in oil
Crab	2 tablespoons crab meat	1.5	
Haddock, smoked	1 fillet	1.5	smoked foods are higher in salt, so limit amounts
Halibut, steamed or grilled	1 fillet	1.5	
Lobster	2 tablespoons	1.5	flavour with lemon juice
Mussels	6 mussels	1.5	
Salmon, smoked	3 slices	1.5	a source of healthy omega-3 fats
Scallops, steamed	3 tablespoons	1.5	
Shrimps	1 teacupful	1.5	
Trout, steamed or grilled	1 fish	1.5	a source of healthy omega-3 fats
Fish fingers, cod, grilled	4 fingers	2	
Herring, grilled	2 fillets	2	a source of healthy omega-3 fats
Salmon, pink, canned in brine, drained	small can	2	a source of healthy omega-3 fats
Salmon, steamed or grilled	1 steak	2	a source of healthy omega-3 fats
Sardines, canned in brine, drained	4 sardines	2	a source of healthy omega-3 fats

Food	Portion Size	GiPs	Special Comments
Kipper, baked	2 fillets	2.5	a source of healthy omega-3 fats, but high in salt
Mackerel, canned in brine, drained	small can	2.5	a source of healthy omega-3 fats

MEATS

Food	Portion Size	GiPs	Special Comments
Beef stew, made with lean beef	2 serving spoons	1.5	limit or avoid fat in cooking
Ham	2 slices	1.5	
Kidney, ox, stewed	3 tablespoons	1.5	
Lamb, loin chops, grilled, lean	2 chops	1.5	
Lamb, scrag and neck, lean only, stewed	2 serving spoons	1.5	limit or avoid fat in cooking
Rabbit, stewed	2 serving spoons	1.5	
Bacon, gammon joint, lean only, cooked	140 g (5 oz) steak	2	cooked weight, high in salt, limit amounts
Beef, sirloin joint, roasted lean	3 slices	2	
Beef, rump steak, lean, grilled	140 g (5 oz) steak	2	cooked weight
Chicken, breast chunks or strips	2 serving spoons	2	
Chicken, roasted	3 slices	2	avoid the skin, breast pieces are lower in fat
Chicken, breast, skinless, roasted	1 medium	2	
Chicken, leg, skinless, roasted	1 medium	2	
Chicken, thigh, skinless, roasted	1 medium	2	
Chicken, wing, skinless, roasted	4 wings	2	see recipe, page 130
Chicken, drumstick, skinless, roasted	2 drumsticks	2	higher in fat than chicken breast
Duck, roasted	3 slices	2	avoid the skin
Kidney, lamb, sautéed	2 kidneys	2	
Liver, ox, stewed	3 tablespoons	2	rich in iron and vitamin B12
Pork, leg joint, roasted	3 slices	2	
Pork, loin chops, grilled, lean	1 chop	2	
Turkey, roasted	2 slices	2	you get three times as much if you use wafer-thin turkey
Beef, mince, stewed	2 serving spoons	2.5	choose lean beef

Food	Portion Size	GiPs	Special Comments
Beef, topside, roasted well-done, lean	3 slices	2.5	
Corned beef, canned	2 slices	2.5	watch the salt!
Lamb, leg joint, roasted, lean	3 slices	2.5	
Lamb, shoulder joint, roasted, lean	3 slices	2.5	
Liver sausage	1 slice	2.5	all sausages tend to be high in salt and very processed
Liver, lamb, sautéed	2 slices	2.5	rich in iron, great for the immune system
Oxtail, stewed	2 serving spoons	2.5	
Tongue, ox, stewed	2 slices	2.5	
Veal, cutlet, sautéed	1 cutlet	2.5	use spray oil
Veal, fillet, roast	1 fillet	2.5	
Bacon rashers, back, grilled	3 rashers	3	GI of turkey rashers is not available, but they are a lower-fat choice
Beef sausages, grilled	2 sausages	3	GI of lower-fat sausages is not available, but they are a better choice
Lamb, breast, roasted, lean	3 slices	3	
Pork sausages, grilled	2 sausages	3	
Bacon rashers, middle, grilled	3 rashers	3.5	
Beefburgers, chilled/frozen, grilled	2 beefburgers	3.5	
Chicken nuggets	6 nuggets	4	

MILK AND DAIRY

Food	Portion Size	GiPs	Special Comments
Soya, non-dairy alternative to milk, unsweetened	200 ml (⅓ pint)	0.5	soy protein is rich in phyto-chemicals, shown to reduce blood cholesterol
Semi-skimmed milk	200 ml (⅓ pint)	0.5	
Skimmed milk	200 ml (⅓ pint)	0.5	
Cottage cheese, plain, reduced-fat	small tub	1	
Custard made with semi-skimmed milk	small yoghurt pot size	1	
Drinking yoghurt	200 ml (⅓ pint)	1	choose reduced calorie if available

Food	Portion Size	GiPs	Special Comments
Flavoured milk, chocolate, reduced-fat	200 ml (⅓ pint)	1	
Strawberry Nesquik made with semi-skimmed milk	200 ml (⅓ pint)	1	GI has been analysed on this brand, but you can choose any brand if you like
Yoghurt, low-fat, natural	small pot	1	
Cheese, ricotta	small tub (150 g/5 oz)	1.5	
Cottage cheese, plain	small tub	1.5	
Chocolate Nesquik made with semi-skimmed milk	200 ml (⅓ pint)	2	
Cheese, Edam-type	small matchbox-size piece	2.5	
Cheese, feta	small matchbox-size piece	2.5	
Cheddar type, half fat	small matchbox-size piece	3	
Mozzarella, fresh	small matchbox-size piece	3	
Cheese, Brie	small matchbox-size piece	3.5	
Cheese, Cheshire	small matchbox-size piece	4	
Cheese, Emmental	small matchbox-size piece	4	
Cheddar cheese	small matchbox-size piece	4.5	grated goes further, use 3 tablespoons
Stilton, blue	small matchbox-size piece	4.5	

NUTS (use nuts in cooking to provide protein)

Food	Portion Size	GiPs	Special Comments
Peanuts, dry roasted	pub pack (25 g/1 oz) or half 50 g pack	3	high in fat but low in saturates and GI, choose nuts once a day strictly in these amounts
Peanuts, roasted and salted	pub pack (25 g/1 oz) or half 50g pack	3	high in fat but low in saturates and GI, choose nuts once a day strictly in these amounts

Food	Portion Size	GiPs	Special Comments
Walnuts	6 halves	3	throw them into salads, choose nuts once a day strictly in these amounts
Almonds	10–12 almonds	3	high in fat but low in GI and saturates, choose nuts once a day strictly in these amounts
Cashew nuts	15 cashews	3.5	high in fat but low in GI, choose nuts once a day strictly in these amounts

VEGETABLES

(packed with free choices)

Food	Portion Size	GiPs
Alfalfa sprouts	as desired	0
Artichoke, globe	as desired	0
Asparagus	as desired	0
Asparagus, canned, drained	as desired	0
Aubergines, grilled	as desired	0
Bamboo shoots, canned, drained	as desired	0
Broccoli, green, frozen, steamed	as desired	0
Broccoli, green, raw	as desired	0
Broccoli, green, steamed	as desired	0
Broccoli, purple sprouting, steamed	as desired	0
Cabbage, spring, steamed	as desired	0
Cabbage, winter, steamed	as desired	0
Cabbage, Chinese, raw	as desired	0
Cabbage, frozen, steamed	as desired	0
Cabbage, red, steamed	as desired	0
Cabbage, Savoy, steamed	as desired	0
Cabbage, summer, steamed	as desired	0
Cabbage, white, steamed	as desired	0
Cauliflower, frozen, steamed	as desired	0
Cauliflower, raw	as desired	0
Cauliflower, steamed	as desired	0
Celeriac, raw	as desired	0

Food	Portion Size	GiPs	Special Comments
Celeriac, steamed	as desired	0	
Celery, raw	as desired	0	
Celery, steamed	as desired	0	
Chard, Swiss, raw	as desired	0	
Chard, Swiss, steamed	as desired	0	
Chicory, raw	as desired	0	
Chicory, steamed	as desired	0	
Courgette, raw	as desired	0	
Courgette, steamed	as desired	0	
Cucumber, raw	as desired	0	
Curly kale, steamed	as desired	0	
Endive, raw	as desired	0	
Fennel, raw	as desired	0	
Fennel, steamed	as desired	0	
Gherkins, pickled, drained	as desired	0	
Gourd, kantola, canned, drained	as desired	0	
Gourd, karela, canned, drained	as desired	0	
Gourd, tinda, canned, drained	as desired	0	
Kohl rabi, raw	as desired	0	
Kohl rabi, steamed	as desired	0	
Leeks, steamed	as desired	0	
Lettuce, butterhead, raw	as desired	0	
Lettuce, Cos, raw	as desired	0	
Lettuce, Iceberg, raw	as desired	0	
Lettuce, mixed leaves	as desired	0	
Lettuce, Webbs, raw	as desired	0	
Lotus tubers, canned	as desired	0	
Marrow, parwal, canned, drained	as desired	0	
Marrow, steamed	as desired	0	
Mushrooms, raw	as desired	0	
Mushrooms, canned, drained	as desired	0	
Mushrooms, oyster, raw	as desired	0	
Mushrooms, steamed	as desired	0	

Food	Portion Size	GiPs	Special Comments
Mushrooms, straw, canned, drained	as desired	0	
Mustard and cress, raw	as desired	0	
Mustard leaves, steamed	as desired	0	
Okra, canned, drained	as desired	0	
Okra, steamed	as desired	0	
Onions, cooked	as desired	0	
Onions, pickled, cocktail/ silverskin, drained	as desired	0	
Peppers, capsicum, steamed	as desired	0	
Peppers, raw	as desired	0	
Raddiccio, raw	as desired	0	
Radish, red, raw	as desired	0	
Radish, white/mooli, raw	as desired	0	
Sauerkraut	as desired	0	
Seakale, steamed	as desired	0	
Shallots, raw	as desired	0	
Spinach, canned, drained	as desired	0	
Spinach, frozen, steamed	as desired	0	
Spinach, raw	as desired	0	
Spinach, steamed	as desired	0	
Spring greens, steamed	as desired	0	
Spring onions, bulbs and tops, raw	as desired	0	
Sweetcorn, baby, canned, drained	as desired	0	
Sweetcorn, baby, fresh and frozen, steamed	as desired	0	
Tomatoes, canned, with juice	as desired	0	make a sauce with onion, garlic and herbs, add to pasta for a low-GiP meal
Tomatoes, cherry, raw	as desired	0	
Tomatoes, raw	as desired	0	
Turnip, steamed	as desired	0	
Vine leaves, preserved in brine	as desired	0	
Watercress, raw	as desired	0	
Brussels sprouts, frozen, steamed	12 sprouts	0.5	

Food	Portion Size	GiPs	Special Comments
Brussels sprouts, steamed	12 sprouts	0.5	
Carrots, fresh, steamed	2 tablespoons	1	
Carrots, frozen, steamed	2 tablespoons	1	
Carrots, young, steamed	2 tablespoons	1	
Courgette, sautéed	1 courgette	1	use spray oil
Haricot beans, dried, steamed	1 teacupful	1	
Butter beans, dried, boiled	1 teacupful	1.5	
Carrot, average raw	1 large carrot	1.5	
Plantain, steamed	1 plantain	1.5	
Seaweed, nori, dried, raw	2 tablespoons	1.5	contains the antioxidant selenium
Yam, baked	size of a medium potato	1.5	
Yam, boiled	size of a medium potato	1.5	
Yam, steamed	size of a medium potato	1.5	
Ackee, canned, drained	½ can	2	
Baked beans, canned in tomato sauce	small can	2	low in GI, high in versatility
Beetroot, pickled, drained	4 slices	2	
Mushrooms, common, stir-fried	2 tablespoons	2	or use a little spray oil and count as 0 GiPs
Peas, fresh, steamed	3 tablespoons	2	
Peas, frozen, steamed	3 tablespoons	2	
Sweetcorn, on-the-cob, whole, steamed	1 cob	2	
Beetroot, cooked	4 slices	2.5	
Cassava, boiled	size of a medium potato	2.5	you can buy cassava frozen in Asian food stores
Cassava, steamed	size of a medium potato	2.5	
Sweetcorn, kernels, canned, drained	3 tablespoons	2.5	choose canned veg in unsalted, unsweetened water
Sweetcorn, kernels, fresh, cooked	3 tablespoons	2.5	
Breadfruit, canned, drained	2 slices	3	

Food	Portion Size	GiPs	Special Comments
Cassava, baked	size of a medium potato	3	
New potatoes, boiled	4 new potatoes	3	keep skins on
New potatoes, canned, drained	4 new potatoes	3	
Old potatoes, boiled	3 egg-size potatoes	3	
Pumpkin, cooked	2 slices	3	
Swede, steamed	2 tablespoons	3	
Sweet potato, boiled	1 small potato	3	
Sweet potato, steamed	1 small potato	3	
Breadfruit, boiled	2 slices	3.5	
Broad beans, boiled	2 tablespoons	3.5	
Sweet potato, baked	1 small potato	3.5	
Matoki, boiled	1 matoki	4	available in African food stores
Chips, straight cut, frozen, oven baked	2 serving spoons	5	choose 5% fat versions
Cassava, gari	1 serving spoon	6	
Chips, French fries, fast food outlet	2 serving spoons	6	
Instant mashed potato made up with water	2 scoops	7	use the same GiP for home-made, add any GiPs from milk or butter
Old potatoes, baked	1 medium potato	7	add a low GiP carb
Parsnip, steamed	2 tablespoons	7	a great veg, but high in GI
Parsnip, roast	2 tablespoons	7.5	

(also see Quick and easy GiP-free snack recipes below)

FRUITS, DESSERTS, SNACKS, DRINKS
(fruits get the gold star)
BAKERY

Currant bun	1 bun	4	
Crumpets	1 crumpet	4	
Currant bread (fruit loaf)	2 slices	4	
Banana bread	1 slice	4.5	
Scotch pancakes	2 pancakes	5	

Food	Portion Size	GiPs	Special Comments
Melba toast, plain	2 toast	7	
Scone plain	1 scone	10	very high GI, hence high point value

BEANS AND LENTILS *(all beans and lentils count once a day as one of your five fruit and veg)*

Chilli beans, canned	½ large can	1	
Baked beans, canned in tomato sauce	small can	2	
Red kidney beans, canned	½ large can	2	
Chick peas, canned	½ large can	2	great spiced up as a snack – add chilli sauce
Broad beans, canned	½ large can	4	

BISCUITS

Rich Tea	2 biscuits	2	
Cream crackers	2 crackers	3	
Crispbread, rye	2 crispbread	3	
Ryvita	2 crispbread	3	
Wholemeal crackers	2 crackers	3	
Oat cakes	2 oat cakes	3.5	use the same GiP for oatmeal biscuits
Rice cakes	2 cakes	7	calories per rice cake are low, but GI is high
Water biscuits	2 biscuits	7.5	calories per biscuit are low, but GI is high

DRINKS

Diet soft drinks	as desired	0	you could go for decaff versions
Water, sparkling	as desired	0	
Water, still	as desired	0	
Water, sugar-free flavoured	as desired	0	check no added sugar
Sugar-free squash	as desired	0	
Tomato juice	1 glass (150 ml)	0	add some Worcester sauce for a bit of zing!

Food	Portion Size	GiPs	Special Comments
Apple juice, unsweetened	1 glass (150 ml)	1.5	cloudy has a slightly lower GI
Grapefruit juice, unsweetened	1 glass (150 ml)	1.5	
Orange juice, unsweetened	1 glass (150 ml)	1.5	
Pineapple juice, unsweetened	1 glass (150 ml)	1.5	
Cranberry juice	1 glass (150 ml)	3	diet versions are lower in calories, but GI value is not available

FRUIT (have five fruit and veg a day: they're rich in antioxidants)

Food	Portion Size	GiPs	Special Comments
Grapefruit	1 grapefruit	0	rich in potassium which helps to regulate blood pressure
Strawberries	1 teacupful	0	keep to portion size if you want to have them GiP-free
Apples	1 apple	0.5	the whole fruit has all the fibre, choose it over fruit juice
Cherries	12 cherries	0.5	
Olives	10 olives	0.5	olives with stones take longer to eat so you might eat less
Peaches, canned in juice	6 slices	0.5	
Pears	1 pear	0.5	
Plums	3 plums	0.5	
Fruit cocktail, canned in juice	½ large can	1	
Kiwi fruit	2 kiwi	1.5	abundant in vitamin C
Oranges	1 large orange	1.5	the GI of satsumas is not available, but you can choose 2–3 satsumas instead of an orange and count the GiPs as 1.5
Peaches	1 peach	1.5	
Pears, canned in juice	2 pear halves	1.5	
Prunes, ready-to-eat	8 prunes	1.5	
Apricots, dried	6 apricots	2	good source of fibre and beta-carotene

Food	Portion Size	GIPs	Special Comments
Bananas	1 small banana	2	great source of potassium
Custard apple	1 custard apple	2	
Dates, dried	4 dates	2	
Grapes	15 grapes	2	
Mangoes	1 small mango	2	
Melon, cantaloupe	½ melon	2	
Apricots, fresh	3 apricots	2.5	
Paw-paw	½ small	2.5	
Pineapple	1 slice	2.5	
Figs, dried	2 figs	3	
Raisins	2 handfuls	3	
Sultanas	2 handfuls	3	
Melon, watermelon	1 slice	3.5	very low in calories but very high in GI

MILK AND DAIRY

Food	Portion Size	GIPs	Special Comments
Soya, non-dairy alternative to milk, unsweetened	200 ml (⅓ pint)	0.5	soy protein is rich in phytochemicals, shown to reduce blood cholesterol
Semi-skimmed milk	200 ml (⅓ pint)	0.5	
Skimmed milk	200 ml (⅓ pint)	0.5	
Custard made with semi-skimmed milk	small yoghurt pot size	1	
Drinking yoghurt	200 ml (⅓ pint)	1	choose reduced calorie if available
Flavoured milk, chocolate, reduced-fat	200 ml (⅓ pint)	1	
Strawberry Nesquik made with semi-skimmed milk	200 ml (⅓ pint)	1	GI has been analysed on this brand, but you can choose any brand if you like
Tzatziki	2 tablespoons	1	opt for lower-fat versions if available
Yoghurt, diet	small pot	1	
Yoghurt, low-fat, natural	small pot	1	
Fromage frais, virtually fat-free	1 pot	1.5	

Food	Portion Size	GiPs	Special Comments
Mousse, reduced-fat	small pot	1.5	
Chocolate Nesquik made with semi-skimmed milk	200 ml (⅓ pint)	2	
Soya, alternative to yoghurt, fruit	small pot	2	
Ice cream, reduced calorie	2 scoops	2.5	

SNACKS (nuts in shells take longer to eat, so you may end up having less)

Food	Portion Size	GiPs	Special Comments
Sesame seeds	2 teaspoons	1	throw them into GiP-free salad for extra crunch
Peanuts, dry roasted	pub pack (25 g/1 oz) or half 50 g pack	3	high in fat but low in GI and saturates, choose nuts once a day strictly in these amounts
Peanuts, roasted and salted	pub pack (25 g/1 oz) or half 50g pack	3	high in fat but low in GI and saturates, choose nuts once a day strictly in these amounts
Walnuts	6 halves	3	high in fat but low in GI and saturates, choose nuts once a day strictly in these amounts
Almonds	10–12 almonds	3	high in fat but low in GI and saturates, choose nuts once a day strictly in these amounts
Cashew nuts	15 cashews	3.5	high in fat but low in GI, choose nuts once a day strictly in these amounts
Popcorn, plain	5 tablespoons	4	choose lower-fat varieties, high GI, see recipe for Chilli Peanut Popcorn. page 133
Cereal chewy bar – dried fruit	45–50 g bar	4.5	
Cereal crunchy bar – dried fruit	45–50 g bar	4.5	
Pretzels	25 g (1 oz) portion	6	a low-fat snack but high in GI

Food	Portion Size	GiPs	Special Comments

SOUPS

Food	Portion Size	GiPs	Special Comments
Minestrone soup, dried, as served	1 soup bowl	0	GI of only these packet soups is available, but you can try other flavours
Tomato soup, dried, as served	1 soup bowl	0.5	
Tomato soup, cream of, canned	1 soup bowl	1	
Instant noodle soup	1 soup bowl	2	
Lentil soup	1 soup bowl	2	

(also see Free Snacks, Breads and Breakfast Cereals for snack ideas)

FREE FLAVOURINGS

(choose as often as you like)

Chilli sauce	0	
Mustard	0	
Soy sauce	0	try low-sodium types
Worcestershire sauce	0	
Vinegar (rice, balsamic, malt, wine)	0	
Oil, spray oil	0	5 sprays per dish, strict portion limit
Dressing, fat-free	0	
Artificial sweeteners	0	
Jelly, sugar-free	0	
Stock cube	0	try low-sodium types
Tomato purée	0	
Herbs, fresh or dried	0	
Spices, fresh (e.g. garlic, ginger, chilli)	0	
Spices, ground (e.g. paprika, chilli powder, curry powder)	0	
Spices, whole (e.g. cumin seeds, coriander seeds, caraway seeds)	0	
Salt	0	keep added salt to a minimum
Salt substitutes	0	
Pepper	0	

Food	Portion Size	GiPs	Special Comments

FATTY AND SUGARY FOODS
(keep to a minimum)

CAKES AND BISCUITS

Food	Portion Size	GiPs	Special Comments
Digestive biscuits, plain	1 biscuit	3.5	reduced-fat versions are available
Muffins, American style, chocolate chip	1 muffin	5	choosing a smaller one means less fat
Muffins, blueberry	1 muffin	5	
Muffins, oat bran	1 muffin	5	
Scotch pancakes	2 pancakes	5	
Danish pastries	small pastry	5.5	
Sponge cake	small slice	6	watch portion size
Croissants	1 croissant	6	
Waffles	1 waffle	6.5	
Doughnuts, ring	1 doughnut	7.5	
Shortbread	2 fingers	7.5	

FATS AND OILS (opt for monounsaturated ones)

Food	Portion Size	GiPs	Special Comments
Spread, low-fat	scraping	0.5	
Spread, half fat, unsaturated	scraping	0.5	some are mono-unsaturated
Spread, very low-fat, unsaturated	1 teaspoon	0.5	
Butter	scraping	1	
Spread, low-fat	1 teaspoon	1	
Spread, half fat, unsaturated	1 teaspoon	1	
Oil, olive oil	1 teaspoon	1.5	monounsaturated
Oil, rapeseed oil	1 teaspoon	1.5	monounsaturated. Also sometimes sold as vegetable oil – check label
Butter	1 teaspoon	2	
Oil, sunflower oil	1 teaspoon	2	if cooking for 4, use 4 tsp and then count your portion as 2 GiPs
Oil, vegetable oil, mixed	1 teaspoon	2	

Food	Portion Size	GIPs	Special Comments

PROCESSED FOODS

Food	Portion Size	GIPs	Special Comments
Bacon rashers, back, grilled	3 rashers	3	GI of turkey rashers is not available, but they are a lower-fat choice
Beef sausages, grilled	2 sausages	3	GI of lower-fat sausages is not available, but they are a better choice
Pork sausages, grilled	2 sausages	3	
Bacon rashers, middle, grilled	3 rashers	3.5	
Beefburgers, chilled/frozen, grilled	2 beefburgers	3.5	
Pizza, cheese and tomato, deep pan	2 slices from medium (9" diameter) or 1 slice of large (12" diameter)	3.5	GI of other pizza toppings not available – if choosing meat toppings, opt for lower-fat types
Pizza, cheese and tomato, thin base	2 slices from medium (9" diameter) or 1 slice of large (12" diameter)	3.5	GI of other pizza toppings not available – avoid extra cheese
Pizza, vegetarian	2 slices from medium (9" diameter) or 1 slice of large (12" diameter)	3.5	choose less cheese and more veggies
Chicken nuggets, takeaway	6 nuggets	4	
Cornish pasty	1 pasty	4	pastry is high in fat
Ice cream, dairy, vanilla	2 scoops	4	
Steak and kidney/Beef pie, individual, chilled/frozen, baked	1 pie	4.5	
Chips, straight cut, frozen, oven baked	2 serving spoons	5	
Chips, French fries, fast food outlet	2 serving spoons	6	
Taco shells, baked	1 shell	7	
Indian pooris	2 pooris	7.5	

CRISPS

Food	Portion Size	GIPs	Special Comments
Corn chips	small packet (30 g)	6	
Potato crisps	small packet (25 g)	6.5	

Food	Portion Size	GiPs	Special Comments

SUGARY FOODS

Food	Portion Size	GiPs	Special Comments
Jam, reduced sugar	1 teaspoon	0.5	
Fructose	2 teaspoons	1	
Honey	1 teaspoon	1	
Jam	1 teaspoon	1	
Marmalade	1 teaspoon	1	
Chocolate, milk	1 square piece	1.5	
Chocolate, milk	1 treat-size bar (15 g)	2	
Chocolate, white	1 treat-size bar (13 g)	2	
Snickers bar	1 fun size (19 g)	2	
Sugar	2 teaspoons	2.5	
Twix	1 mini Twix (21 g)	2.5	
Mars bar	1 fun size (19 g)	3	
Candies, jellybeans	6 jelly beans	4	
Nougat	4 sweets	4	
Chocolate-covered peanuts (e.g. M&M)	1 small pack (47 g/2 oz)	5	
Sparkling glucose drink	1 glass (150 ml)	7	
Glucose – liquid	2 teaspoons	9.5	goes straight into the blood stream!

GO LOW WITH A COMBO

(made-up healthy choices that can save you GiPs.
You could add a fruit or fruit juice to provide balance)

BREAKFAST CHOICES

	GiPs	
Peanut butter (2 tsp) on 1 slice of wholemeal bread	3.5	no other nuts allowed on the same day. GI for peanut butter on its own is not available
Burgen soya and linseed bread (2 slices) with low-fat spread (scraping) and Edam cheese (small matchbox-size piece)	4	
Oat cakes (2) with low-fat spread (scraping) and plain cottage cheese (small tub)	5	

Food	Portion Size	GiPs	Special Comments
Wholemeal bread (2 slices) with low-fat spread (scraping) and banana (1)		6	
Granary bread (2 slices) with scrambled egg (2) and tomato		6	
Wholemeal bread (2 slices) with butter (1 tsp) and poached eggs (2)		8	

LUNCH CHOICES

Food	Portion Size	GiPs	Special Comments
Burgen soya and linseed bread (2 slices) with low-fat spread (1 tsp), tuna (small can) and cucumber		3	
Wheat tortilla (1) with chicken (3 slices) and mixed green salad		4	
Wheat tortilla (1) with mozzarella cheese (small matchbox-size piece, chopped), beef tomato and basil		4.5	
Granary bread (2 slices) with low-fat spread (1 tsp), ham (2 slices) and salad		5	
Granary bread (2 slices) with low-fat spread (1 tsp), mozzarella cheese (1 slice), fresh basil and tomato		5.5	
Pumpernickel bread (2 slices) and low-fat spread (1 tsp), ham (2 slices), mixed green salad		5.5	
Jacket potato with low-fat spread (1 tsp), cottage cheese (small tub) and sliced peppers		6.5	
Wholemeal bread (2 slices) with low-fat spread (1 tsp), cottage cheese (small tub) and shredded cucumber and lettuce		6.5	
Jacket potato with low-fat spread (1 tsp), tuna (small can) and sweetcorn (3 tablespoons)		7	
Wholemeal bread (2 slices) with low-fat spread (1 tsp), melted Edam (1 slice) and tomato		7	
Jacket potato with low-fat spread (1 tsp), half-fat Cheddar cheese (3 tablespoons, grated) and side salad (fat-free dressing)		9.5	
Baguette (1 small) with low-fat spread (1 tsp), prawns (small jar) and mixed green salad (fat-free dressing)		10.5	
Baguette (1 small) with low-fat spread (1 tsp), roast beef (3 slices), lettuce and mustard		12	

Food	Portion Size	GiPs	Special Comments

THE RECIPES
(see Chapter 8)

MAIN MEALS

Food		GiPs	
Cod Kebabs with Fresh Dill		1.5	
Sizzling Turkey Burgers		1.5	
Turkey Stroganoff		1.5	
Herby Pork Chops		2	
Haddock with Thai Green Pepper and Basil Sauce		2.5	
Cheesy Pork Chops		2.5	
Sweet and Sour Chicken Drumsticks		3	
Salmon Steaks in Garlicky Balsamic Vinegar		3.5	
Couscous with Peppers and Red Onion		4.5	
Mediterranean Pasta		5	
Instant Noodles with Prawns and Garlic		6.5	
Beef Chow Mein		7	

STARTERS AND SIDES

Food		GiPs	Special Comments
Baked Tiger Prawns		1	
Beef Tomatoes with Black Olives		1	
Curried Cauliflower		1	
Layered Mushroom and Tomato with Grilled Cheese		1	
Chilli and Honey Chicken Wings		2	
Char-grilled Vegetables with Honey and Basil		2	
Chilli Peanut Popcorn		2.5	no other nuts or peanut butter allowed on the same day
Kidney Bean and Chick Pea Salad in Mustard Dressing		2.5	
Middle Eastern Tabouleh Salad		3	

Food	Portion Size	GiPs	Special Comments

SPEEDY GIP-FREE SNACK RECIPES (see page 151)

Food		GiPs
Garlic Mushrooms		0
Cabbage with Fennel Seeds		0
Grilled Tomato Salad		0
Courgette Boats		0
Chilli and Lime Rocket Leaves		0
Warming Marrow and Leek Soup		0
Savoy Cabbage with Caraway Seeds		0
Herby Baby Spinach and Beansprouts		0
Gherkin and Onion Pickle		0
Stir-fried Babycorn		0
Curried Okra		0
Balsamic French Beans		0
Hot Roasted Vegetables		0
Speedy Salsa Sauce		0
Cucumber and Mint Cooler		0
Spiced Vegetables		0
Al Dente Asparagus		0
Wheat-free Tabouleh		0
Jelly with Whole Strawberries		0

(also see Vegetables for 'free' snack ideas)

READY MEALS

Food	Portion Size	GiPs	Special Comments
Instant gravy	2 serving spoons	0.5	can be high in salt, but lower in fat than using meat juices
Quorn, pieces, as purchased	12 pieces	1	a great low-fat meat substitute, use the same GiP for two Quorn burgers
Ravioli, meat	12 ravioli	1.5	
Indian Dhokra	4 pieces	2	
Sushi	6 mini	2.5	

Food	Portion Size	GIPs	Special Comments
Tortellini, cheese	12 tortellini	3	remember to add any points from sauces
Vine leaves, stuffed with rice	8 medium vine leaves	3	
Beans, mung, green, gram, cooked dahl	1 teacupful	3.5	use as little oil as possible if cooking from scratch
Lamb/Beef hot pot with potatoes, chilled/frozen	ready meal portion	3.5	look out for supermarket healthier versions
Pizza, cheese and tomato, deep pan	2 slices from medium (9" diameter) or 1 slice of large (12" diameter)	3.5	GI of other pizza toppings not available – if choosing meat toppings, opt for lower-fat types
Pizza, cheese and tomato, thin base	2 slices from medium (9" diameter) or 1 slice of large (12" diameter)	3.5	GI of other pizza toppings not available – avoid extra cheese
Pizza, vegetarian	2 slices from medium (9" diameter) or 1 slice of large (12" diameter)	3.5	choose less cheese and more veggies
Chicken nuggets, takeaway	6 nuggets	4	
Cornish pasty	1 pasty	4	pastry is high in fat, go easy
Macaroni cheese	2 serving spoons	4	tomato-based sauces tend to be lower in calories and richer in antioxidants
Chicken, stir-fried with rice and vegetables, frozen	ready meal portion	4.5	
Steak and kidney/Beef pie, individual, chilled/frozen, baked	1 pie	4.5	

Food	Portion Size	GiPs	Special Comments

ALPHABETICAL POINT TABLE

BEANS AND LENTILS *all beans and lentils count once a day as one of your five fruit and veg. These are also protein foods and if you choose them as your protein, then choose another meal carb*

FATS AND OILS *opt for monounsaturated ones and keep to a minimum*

FRUIT *have five fruit and veg a day, they're rich in antioxidants*

FISH *choose fish twice a week, one being oily fish which is rich in omega-3 fats*

NUTS *nuts in shells take longer to eat, which may help you have less when snacking*

PASTA *add GiPs from sauces. Use 50 g (2 oz) raw per portion*

RICE AND GRAINS *keep rice grains whole rather than soft and mushy*

VEGETABLES *some of these are part of meal carbs since they are high in starch*

A

Food	Portion Size	GiPs	Special Comments
Ackee, canned, drained	½ can	2	
Alfalfa sprouts	as desired	0	
Apples	1 apple	0.5	the whole fruit has all the fibre, choose it over fruit juice
Apricots, dried	6 apricots	2	good source of fibre and beta-carotene
Apricots, fresh	3 apricots	2.5	
Artichoke, globe	as desired	0	
Artificial sweeteners	as desired	0	
Asparagus	as desired	0	
Asparagus, canned, drained	as desired	0	
Aubergines, grilled	as desired	0	

B

Food	Portion Size	GiPs	Special Comments
Bacon rashers, back, grilled	3 rashers	3	GI of turkey rashers is not available, but they are a lower-fat choice
Bacon rashers, middle, grilled	3 rashers	3.5	

Food	Portion Size	GiPs	Special Comments
Bacon, gammon joint, lean only, cooked	5 oz steak	2	cooked weight, high in salt, limit amounts
Beans, baked, canned in tomato sauce	small can	2	low in GI, high in versatility
Bamboo shoots, canned, drained	as desired	0	
Banana bread	1 slice	4.5	
Bananas	1 small banana	2	great source of potassium
Barley, pearl, cooked	1 teacupful	1.5	throw some into soups and stews
Beans, mung, green, gram, cooked dahl	1 teacupful	3.5	use as little oil as possible if cooking from scratch
Beans, blackeye, dried, cooked	1 teacupful	1.5	
Beans, broad, canned	½ large can	4	
Beans, broad, dried, cooked	1 teacupful	3.5	
Beans, broad, frozen, cooked	1 teacupful	4	
Beans, butter beans, dried, cooked	1 teacupful	1.5	
Beans, chilli, canned	½ large can	1	
Beans, haricot, dried, cooked	1 teacupful	1	
Beans, haricot, dried, steamed	1 teacupful	1	
Beans, mung, whole, dried, cooked	1 teacupful	2	
Beans, pinto, dried, cooked	1 teacupful	1.5	
Beans, red kidney, canned	½ large can	2	
Beans, red kidney, dried, cooked	1 teacupful	1.5	you can use a combination of beans in smaller portions for the same points
Beef sausages, grilled	2 sausages	3	GI of lower-fat sausages is not available, but they are a better choice
Beef, sirloin joint, roasted, lean	3 slices	2	
Beef stew, made with lean beef	2 serving spoons	1.5	limit or avoid fat in cooking
Beef, mince, stewed	2 serving spoons	2.5	choose lean beef
Beef, rump steak, lean, grilled	5 oz steak	2	cooked weight
Beef, topside, roasted well-done, lean	3 slices	2.5	
Beefburgers, chilled/frozen, grilled	2 beefburgers	3.5	

Food	Portion Size	GiPs	Special Comments
Beetroot, cooked	4 slices	2.5	
Beetroot, pickled, drained	4 slices	2	
Biscuits, cream crackers	2 crackers	3	
Biscuits, crispbread, rye	2 crispbreads	3	
Biscuits, digestive, plain	1 biscuit	3.5	reduced-fat versions are available
Biscuits, oat cakes	2 oat cakes	3.5	use the same GiP for oatmeal biscuits
Biscuits, rice cakes	2 cakes	7	calories per rice cake are low, but GI is high
Biscuits, Rich Tea	2 biscuits	2	
Biscuits, Ryvita	2 crispbreads	3	
Biscuits, shortbread	2 fingers	7.5	
Biscuits, water	2 biscuits	7.5	calories per biscuit are low, but GI is high
Biscuits, wholemeal crackers	2 crackers	3	
Bread, bagels, plain	1 bagel	6	a low-GiP carb filling (e.g. vegetables) helps to reduce the GI of the meal
Bread, baguette	1 individual	9	a great food but a very high GI. Eat always with a low GiP carb filling (e.g. sweetcorn)
Bread, barley	2 slices	3	
Bread, barley and sunflower	2 slices	4.5	
Bread, Burgen oat bran, barley and honey	2 slices	2.5	
Bread, Burgen soya and linseed	2 slices	2.5	grains and seeds tend to lower the GI
Bread, granary	2 slices	3.5	
Bread, hamburger buns	1 bun	5	
Bread, Hovis	2 slices	5.5	
Bread, Melba toast, plain	2 toasts	7	
Bread, mixed grain	2 slices	3.5	wholegrains are richer in B vitamins than refined grains
Bread, pitta	1 pitta	5	wholemeal ones are higher in fibre

Food	Portion Size	GiPs	Special Comments
Bread, pumpernickel	2 slices	3.5	
Bread, rye	2 slices	4.5	
Bread, white	2 slices	5.5	
Bread, white, with added fibre	2 slices	4.5	
Bread, wholemeal	2 slices	5.5	opt for stoneground as it is more coarse and thus has a lower GI
Breadfruit, boiled	2 slices	3.5	
Breadfruit, canned, drained	2 slices	3	
Breakfast cereals			*see Cereal*
Broccoli, green, frozen, steamed	as desired	0	
Broccoli, green, raw	as desired	0	
Broccoli, green, steamed	as desired	0	
Broccoli, purple sprouting, steamed	as desired	0	
Brussels sprouts, frozen, steamed	12 sprouts	0.5	
Brussels sprouts, steamed	12 sprouts	0.5	
Bulgur, cooked	1 teacupful	2	
Butter	scraping	1	
Butter	1 teaspoon	2	

C

Food	Portion Size	GiPs	Special Comments
Cabbage, spring, steamed	as desired	0	
Cabbage, winter, steamed	as desired	0	
Cabbage, Chinese, raw	as desired	0	
Cabbage, frozen, steamed	as desired	0	
Cabbage, red, steamed	as desired	0	
Cabbage, Savoy, steamed	as desired	0	
Cabbage, summer, steamed	as desired	0	
Cabbage, white, steamed	as desired	0	
Candies, jellybeans	6 jelly beans	4	
Carrot, average, raw	1 large carrot	1.5	
Carrots, fresh, steamed	2 tablespoons	1	
Carrots, frozen, steamed	2 tablespoons	1	

Food	Portion Size	GiPs	Special Comments
Carrots, young, steamed	2 tablespoons	1	
Cassava, baked	size of a medium potato	3	
Cassava, boiled	size of a medium potato	2.5	you can buy cassava frozen in Asian shops
Cassava, gari	1 serving spoon	6	
Cassava, steamed	size of a medium potato	2.5	
Cauliflower, frozen, steamed	as desired	0	
Cauliflower, raw	as desired	0	
Cauliflower, steamed	as desired	0	
Celeriac, raw	as desired	0	
Celeriac, steamed	as desired	0	
Celery, raw	as desired	0	
Celery, steamed	as desired	0	
Cereal bar, chewy – dried fruit	45–50 g bar	4.5	
Cereal bar, crunchy – dried fruit	45–50 g bar	4.5	
Cereal, All Bran and semi-skimmed milk	5 tablespoons+ 200 ml (⅓ pint)	2	try it with sliced banana
Cereal, Bran Flakes and semi-skimmed milk	4 tablespoons+ 200 ml (⅓ pint)	4	
Cereal, Cornflakes and semi-skimmed milk	5 tablespoons+ 200 ml (⅓ pint)	4.5	
Cereal, Grapenuts and semi-skimmed milk	5 tablespoons+ 200 ml (⅓ pint)	4.5	
Cereal, instant hot oats made with semi-skimmed milk	follow pack instructions using 200 ml (⅓ pint) milk	4.5	a sachet at work could be a convenient breakfast
Cereal, muesli and semi-skimmed milk	3 tablespoons+ 200 ml (⅓ pint)	4	
Cereal, muesli, reduced sugar and semi-skimmed milk	3 tablespoons+ 200 ml (⅓ pint)	4	
Cereal, muesli, Swiss-style, and semi-skimmed milk	3 tablespoons+ 200 ml (⅓ pint)	4	
Cereal, Nutrigrain and semi-skimmed milk	5 tablespoons+ 200 ml (⅓ pint)	4.5	

Food	Portion Size	GiPs	Special Comments
Cereal, porridge, made with milk and water	6 tablespoons of made-up porridge using 100 ml milk and water as required	3.5	you could try skimmed milk, 200 ml (⅓ pint), instead. Use a little sweetener, honey or fructose if you like, add the GiPs
Cereal, porridge, made with water	8 tablespoons of made-up porridge as per pack instructions	3	
Cereal, Puffed Wheat and semi-skimmed milk	5 tablespoons+ 200 ml (⅓ pint)	4	
Cereal, Raisin Splitz and semi-skimmed milk	4 tablespoons+ 200 ml (⅓ pint)	4.5	
Cereal, Rice Krispies and semi-skimmed milk	7 tablespoons+ 200 ml (⅓ pint)	5.5	
Cereal, Shredded Wheat and semi-skimmed milk	2 biscuits+ 200 ml (⅓ pint)	4.5	
Cereal, Special K and semi-skimmed milk	5 tablespoons+ 200 ml (⅓ pint)	4	
Cereal, Sultana Bran and semi-skimmed milk	4 tablespoons+ 200 ml (⅓ pint)	4.5	
Cereal, Weetabix and semi-skimmed milk	2 biscuits+ 200 ml (⅓ pint)	4.5	
(also see Combo Breakfast Choices, page 83)			
Chapatis, made with fat	2 small chapatis	5.5	
Chapatis, made without fat	2 small chapatis	4.5	use coarse wholemeal chapati flour
Chard, Swiss, raw	as desired	0	
Chard, Swiss, steamed	as desired	0	
Cheese, Brie	small matchbox-size piece	3.5	
Cheese, Cheddar	small matchbox-size piece	4.5	grated goes further, use 3 tablespoons
Cheese, Cheddar type, half fat	small matchbox-size piece	3	
Cheese, Cheshire	small matchbox-size piece	4	
Cheese, cottage cheese, plain	small tub	1.5	

Food	Portion Size	GiPs	Special Comments
Cheese, cottage cheese, plain, reduced-fat	small tub	1	
Cheese, Edam-type	small matchbox-size piece	2.5	
Cheese, Emmental	small matchbox-size piece	4	
Cheese, feta	small matchbox-size piece	2.5	
Cheese, mozzarella, fresh	small matchbox-size piece	3	
Cheese, ricotta	small tub (150 g)	1.5	
Cheese, Stilton, blue	small matchbox-size piece	4.5	
Cherries	12 cherries	0.5	
Chick peas, canned	½ large can	2	great spiced up as a snack – add chilli sauce
Chick peas, split, dried, cooked	1 teacupful	2.5	
Chick peas, whole, dried, cooked	1 teacupful	1.5	
Chicken nuggets, takeaway	6 nuggets	4	
Chicken, breast chunks or strips	2 serving spoons	2	
Chicken, breast, skinless, roasted	1 medium	2	
Chicken, drumstick, skinless, roasted	2 drumsticks	2	chicken breast is lower in fat
Chicken, leg, skinless, roasted	1 medium	2	
Chicken, roasted	3 slices	2	avoid the skin, breast pieces are lower in fat
Chicken, stir-fried with rice and vegetables, frozen	ready meal portion	4.5	
Chicken, thigh, skinless, roasted	1 medium	2	
Chicken, wing, skinless, roasted	4 wings	2	see recipe page 130
Chicory, raw	as desired	0	
Chicory, steamed	as desired	0	
Chilli sauce	as desired	0	
Chips, French fries, fast food outlet	2 serving spoons	6	
Chips, straight cut, frozen, oven baked	2 serving spoons	5	choose 5% fat varieties

Food	Portion Size	GiPs	Special Comments
Chocolate-covered peanuts (e.g. M&M)	1 small pack (47 g)	5	
Chocolate, milk	1 square piece	1.5	
Chocolate, milk	1 treat-size bar (15 g)	2	
Chocolate, white	1 treat-size bar (13 g)	2	
Cockles	6 cockles	1	
Cod, baked	1 fillet	1	
Cod, grilled	1 fillet	1	
Corn chips	small packet (30 g)	6	
Corned beef, canned	2 slices	2.5	watch the salt!
Cornish pasty	1 pasty	4	pastry is high in fat
Courgette, raw	as desired	0	
Courgette, sauted	1 courgette	1	see recipe for GiP-free courgette boats
Courgette, steamed	as desired	0	
Couscous, cooked	1 teacupful	3.5	a nice change from rice
Crab	2 tablespoons crab meat	1.5	
Crisps, potato	small packet (25 g)	6.5	
Croissants	1 croissant	6	
Crumpets	1 crumpet	4	
Cucumber, raw	as desired	0	
Curly kale, steamed	as desired	0	
Currant bread (fruit loaf)	2 slices	4	
Currant bun	1 bun	4	
Custard apple	1 custard apple	2	
Custard, made with semi-skimmed milk	small yoghurt pot size	1	

D

Danish pastries	small pastry	5.5	
Dates, dried	4 dates	2	

Food	Portion Size	GiPs	Special Comments
Dhokra, Indian	4 pieces	2	
Diet soft drinks	as desired	0	you could go for decaff versions
Doughnuts, ring	1 doughnut	7.5	
Dressing, fat-free	as desired	0	avoid added sugar
Drinking yoghurt	200 ml (⅓ pint)	1	choose reduced calorie if available
Duck, roasted	3 slices	2	avoid the skin

E

Food	Portion Size	GiPs	Special Comments
Eggs, boiled	2 eggs	1.5	
Eggs, fried	2 eggs	3	
Eggs, poached	2 eggs	1.5	
Eggs, scrambled, with milk and 1 tsp oil	2 eggs	3	
Endive, raw	as desired	0	

F

Food	Portion Size	GiPs	Special Comments
Fennel, raw	as desired	0	
Fennel, steamed	as desired	0	
Figs, dried	2 figs	3	
Fish fingers, cod, grilled	4 fingers	2	
Fromage frais, virtually fat-free	1 pot	1.5	
Fructose	2 teaspoons	1	
Fruit cocktail, canned in juice	½ large can	1	
Fruit loaf			*see Currant bread*

G

Food	Portion Size	GiPs	Special Comments
Gherkins, pickled, drained	as desired	0	
Glucose – liquid	2 teaspoons	9.5	goes straight into the blood stream!
Gourd, kantola, canned, drained	as desired	0	
Gourd, karela, canned, drained	as desired	0	
Gourd, tinda, canned, drained	as desired	0	

Food	Portion Size	GiPs	Special Comments
Grapefruit	1 grapefruit	0	rich in potassium which helps to regulate blood pressure
Grapefruit juice, unsweetened	1 glass (150 ml)	1.5	
Grapes	15 grapes	2	
Gravy, instant	2 serving spoons	0.5	can be high in salt, but lower in fat than using meat juices
H			
Haddock, smoked	1 fillet	1.5	smoked foods are higher in salt, so limit amounts
Haddock, steamed or grilled	1 fillet	1	
Halibut, steamed or grilled	1 fillet	1.5	
Ham	2 slices	1.5	
Herbs, fresh or dried	as desired	0	
Herring, grilled	2 fillets	2	a source of healthy omega-3 fats
Honey	1 teaspoon	1	
I			
Ice cream, dairy, vanilla	2 scoops	4	
Ice cream, reduced calorie	2 scoops	2.5	
J			
Jam	1 teaspoon	1	
Jam, reduced sugar	1 teaspoon	0.5	
Jelly, sugar-free	as desired	0	
Juice, apple, unsweetened	1 glass (150 ml)	1.5	cloudy has a slightly lower GI
Juice, cranberry	1 glass (150 ml)	3	diet versions are lower in calories, but GI value is not available
Juice, grapefruit, unsweetened	1 glass (150 ml)	1.5	
Juice, orange, unsweetened	1 glass (150 ml)	1.5	
Juice, pineapple, unsweetened	1 glass (150 ml)	1.5	
Juice, tomato	1 glass (150 ml)	0	add some Worcester sauce for a bit of zing!

Food	Portion Size	GiPs	Special Comments
K			
Kidney, lamb, sautéed	2 kidneys	2	
Kidney, ox, stewed	3 tablespoons	1.5	
Kipper, baked	2 fillets	2.5	a source of healthy omega-3 fats, but high in salt
Kiwi fruit	2 kiwi	1.5	abundant in vitamin C
Kohl rabi, raw	as desired	0	
Kohl rabi, steamed	as desired	0	
L			
Lamb, leg joint, roasted, lean	3 slices	2.5	
Lamb, loin chops, grilled, lean	2 chops	1.5	
Lamb, shoulder joint, roasted, lean	3 slices	2.5	
Lamb, breast, roasted, lean	3 slices	3	
Lamb, scrag and neck, lean only, stewed	2 serving spoons	1.5	limit or avoid fat in cooking
Lamb/Beef hot pot with potatoes, chilled/frozen	ready meal portion	3.5	look out for supermarket healthier versions
Leeks, steamed	as desired	0	
Lemon sole, steamed or grilled	1 fillet	1	
Lentils, black gram, urad gram, dried, cooked	1 teacupful	2	
Lentils, red, split, dried, cooked	1 teacupful	1	
Lettuce, butterhead, raw	as desired	0	
Lettuce, Cos, raw	as desired	0	
Lettuce, Iceberg, raw	as desired	0	
Lettuce, mixed leaves	as desired	0	
Lettuce, Webbs, raw	as desired	0	
Liver sausage	1 slice	2.5	all sausages tend to be high in salt and very processed
Liver, lamb, sautéed	2 slices	2.5	rich in iron, great for the immune system
Liver, ox, stewed	3 tablespoons	2	rich in iron and vitamin B12

Food	Portion Size	GiPs	Special Comments
Lobster	2 tablespoons	1.5	
Lotus tubers, canned	as desired	0	

M

Food	Portion Size	GiPs	Special Comments
Mackerel, canned in brine, drained	small can	2.5	a source of healthy omega-3 fats
Mangoes	1 small mango	2	
Marmalade	1 teaspoon	1	
Marrow, parwal, canned, drained	as desired	0	
Marrow, steamed	as desired	0	
Mars bar	1 fun size (19 g)	3	
Matoki, boiled	1 matoki	4	available from Asian/West Indian shops
Melon, cantaloupe	½ melon	2	
Melon, watermelon	1 slice	3.5	very low in calories but very high in GI
Milk, flavoured, Chocolate Nesquik made with semi-skimmed milk	200 ml (⅓ pint)	2	
Milk,, flavoured, chocolate, reduced-fat	200 ml (⅓ pint)	1	
Milk, flavoured, Strawberry Nesquik made with semi-skimmed milk	200 ml (⅓ pint)	1	GI has been analysed on this brand, but you can choose any brand if you like
Milk, semi-skimmed	200 ml (⅓ pint)	0.5	
Milk, skimmed	200 ml (⅓ pint)	0.5	
Mousse, reduced-fat	small pot	1.5	
Muffins, American style, chocolate chip	1 muffin	5	choosing a smaller one means less fat
Muffins, blueberry	1 muffin	5	
Muffins, oat bran	1 muffin	5	
Mushrooms, raw	as desired	0	
Mushrooms, canned, drained	as desired	0	
Mushrooms, common, stir-fried	2 tablespoons	2	use 5 sprays instead of oil and count as 0
Mushrooms, oyster, raw	as desired	0	

Food	Portion Size	GiPs	Special Comments
Mushrooms, steamed	as desired	0	
Mushrooms, straw, canned, drained	as desired	0	
Mussels	6 mussels	1.5	
Mustard	as desired	0	
Mustard and cress, raw	as desired	0	
Mustard leaves, steamed	as desired	0	

N

Food	Portion Size	GiPs	Special Comments
Nougat	4 sweets	4	
Nuts, almonds	10–12 almonds	3	high in fat but low in GI and saturates, choose nuts once a day strictly in these amounts
Nuts, cashews	15 cashews	3.5	high in fat but low in GI, choose nuts once a day strictly in these amounts
Nuts, peanuts, dry roasted	pub pack (25 g/1 oz) or half 50g pack	3	high in fat but low in GI and saturates, choose nuts once a day strictly in these amounts
Nuts, peanuts, roasted and salted	pub pack (25 g/1 oz) or half 50g pack	3	high in fat but low in GI and saturates, choose nuts once a day strictly in these amounts
Nuts, walnuts	6 halves	3	high in fat but low in saturates and GI, choose nuts once a day strictly in these amounts

O

Food	Portion Size	GiPs	Special Comments
Oat cakes			*see Biscuits*
Oil, olive oil	1 teaspoon	1.5	monounsaturated
Oil, rapeseed oil	1 teaspoon	1.5	monounsaturated. Also sometimes sold as vegetable oil – check label
Oil, spray oil	5 sprays per dish	0	strict portion limit
Oil, sunflower oil	1 teaspoon	2	if cooking for 4, use 4 teaspoons and then count your portion as 2 GiPs

Food	Portion Size	GiPs	Special Comments
Oil, vegetable oil, mixed	1 teaspoon	2	
Okra, canned, drained	as desired	0	
Okra, steamed	as desired	0	
Olives	10 olives	0.5	olives with stones take longer to eat so you eat less!
Omelette, plain, made with 1 tsp oil	2 eggs	3	
Onions, cooked	as desired	0	
Onions, pickled, cocktail/silverskin, drained	as desired	0	
Oranges	1 large orange	1.5	the GI of satsumas is not available, but you can choose 2–3 satsumas instead of an orange and count the GiPs as 1.5
Oxtail, stewed	2 serving spoons	2.5	
Oysters	1 dozen oysters	1	shellfish are a good source of zinc, great for immune function

P

Food	Portion Size	GiPs	Special Comments
Parsnip, boiled	2 tablespoons	7	serve with low-GiP vegetables
Parsnip, roast	2 tablespoons	7.5	
Parsnip, steamed	2 tablespoons	7	a great veg, but high in GI
Pasta, fettucini, egg, cooked	5 tablespoons	1.5	
Pasta, linguini, thick, cooked	5 tablespoons	2.5	
Pasta, linguini, thin, cooked	5 tablespoons	2.5	
Pasta, macaroni cheese	2 serving spoons	4	tomato-based sauces tend to be lower in calories and richer in antioxidants
Pasta, macaroni, cooked	5 tablespoons	2	
Pasta, noodles, instant, cooked	5 tablespoons	2	
Pasta, noodles, rice, cooked	5 tablespoons	3	
Pasta, plain, cooked	5 tablespoons	3	
Pasta, ravioli, meat	12 ravioli	1.5	
Pasta, spaghetti, white, cooked	5 tablespoons	1.5	use 50 g/2 oz raw

Food	Portion Size	GIPs	Special Comments
Pasta, spaghetti, wholemeal, cooked	5 tablespoons	1.5	
Pasta, tortellini, cheese	12 tortellini	3	remember to add any points from sauces
Paw-paw	½ small	2.5	
Peaches	1 peach	1.5	
Peaches, canned in juice	6 slices	0.5	
Pears	1 pear	0.5	
Pears, canned in juice	2 pear halves	1.5	
Peas, fresh, steamed	3 tablespoons	2	
Pepper, whole or ground	as desired	0	
Peppers, capsicum, steamed	as desired	0	
Peppers, raw	as desired	0	
Pigeon peas, whole, dried, cooked	1 teacupful	1.5	
Pineapple	1 slice	2.5	
Pineapple juice, unsweetened	1 glass (150 ml)	1.5	
Pizza, cheese and tomato, deep pan	2 slices from medium (9" diameter) or 1 slice of large (12" diameter)	3.5	GI of other pizza toppings not available – avoid extra cheese
Pizza, cheese and tomato, thin base	2 slices from medium (9" diameter) or 1 slice of large (12" diameter)	3.5	GI of other pizza toppings not available – if choosing meat toppings, opt for lower-fat types
Pizza, vegetarian	2 slices from medium (9" diameter) or 1 slice of large (12" diameter)	3.5	choose less cheese and more veggies
Plaice, steamed or grilled	1 fillet	1	
Plantain, boiled	1 plantain	1.5	available from West Indian shops
Plantain, steamed	1 plantain	1.5	
Plums	3 plums	0.5	
Pooris, Indian	2 pooris	7.5	deep fried, so have on occasions only

Food	Portion Size	GiPs	Special Comments
Popcorn, plain	5 tablespoons	4	choose lower-fat varieties, high GI
Pork, leg joint, roasted	3 slices	2	
Pork sausages, grilled	2 sausages	3	
Pork, loin chops, grilled, lean	1 chop	2	
Potato, instant mashed, made up with water	2 scoops	7	use the same GiP for home-made, add any GiPs from milk or butter
Potatoes, new, boiled	4 new potatoes	3	
Potatoes, new, canned, drained	4 new potatoes	3	
Potatoes, old, baked	1 medium potato	7	serve with a low-GiP carb such as baked beans and salad
Potatoes, old, boiled	3 egg-size potatoes	3	
Prawns	1 small jar	1	if you need a dressing, choose fat-free types
Pretzels	25 g portion	6	a low-fat snack but high in GI
Prunes, ready-to-eat	8 prunes	1.5	
Pumpkin, cooked	2 slices	3	

Q

Quorn, pieces, as purchased	12 pieces	1	a great low-fat meat substitute, use the same GiP for two Quorn burgers

R

Rabbit, stewed	2 serving spoons	1.5	
Raddiccio, raw	as desired	0	
Radish leaves, raw	as desired	0	
Radish, red, raw	as desired	0	
Radish, white/mooli, raw	as desired	0	
Raisins	2 handfuls	3	
Rice, brown, boiled	2 serving spoons	2.5	
Rice, white, Bangladeshi, boiled	2 serving spoons	1.5	available from Asian grocers
Rice, white, basmati, boiled	2 serving spoons	2.5	

Food	Portion Size	GiPs	Special Comments
Rice, white, easy cook, boiled	2 serving spoons	3	
Rice, white, glutinous (sticky), boiled	2 serving spoons	7	
Rice, white, instant, boiled	2 serving spoons	3.5	
Rice, white, jasmine, boiled	2 serving spoons	7.5	
Rice, white, polished, boiled	2 serving spoons	3.5	
Rice, white, precooked, microwaved	2 serving spoons	2.5	
Rice, white, risotto, boiled	2 serving spoons	3.5	

S

Food	Portion Size	GiPs	Special Comments
Salmon, pink, canned in brine, drained	small can	2	a source of healthy omega-3 fats
Salmon, smoked	3 slices	1.5	a source of healthy omega-3 fats
Salmon, steamed or grilled	1 steak	2	a source of healthy omega-3 fats
Salt	sprinkling	0	keep added salt to a minimum
Salt substitutes	as desired	0	
Sardines, canned in brine, drained	4 sardines	2	a source of healthy omega-3 fats
Sauerkraut	as desired	0	
Scallops, steamed	3 tablespoons	1.5	
Scone, plain	1 scone	10	very high GI, hence high points value
Scotch pancakes	2 pancakes	5	
Seakale, steamed	as desired	0	
Seaweed, nori, dried, raw	2 tablespoons	1.5	contains the antioxidant selenium
Semolina, cooked, dry	1 teacupful	4.5	
Sesame seeds	2 teaspoons	1	throw them into GiP-free salad for extra crunch
Shallots, raw	as desired	0	
Shrimps	1 teacupful	1.5	
Shrimps, canned in brine, drained	1 small pot	1	

Food	Portion Size	GiPs	Special Comments
Snickers bar	1 fun size (19 g)	2	
Soup, instant noodle	1 soup bowl	2	
Soup, lentil	1 soup bowl	2	
Soup, minestrone, dried, as served	1 soup bowl	0	GI of only these packet soups is available, but you can try other flavours
Soup, tomato, cream of, canned	1 soup bowl	1	
Soup, tomato, dried, as served	1 soup bowl	0.5	
Soy sauce	small amounts	0	try low-sodium types
Soya beans, dried, cooked	1 teacupful	1.5	GI of some canned beans is not available
Soya, alternative to yoghurt, fruit	small pot	2	
Soya, non-dairy alternative to milk, unsweetened	200 ml (⅓ pint)	0.5	soy protein is rich in phytochemicals, shown to reduce blood cholesterol
Sparkling glucose drink	1 glass (150 ml)	7	
Spices, fresh (e.g. garlic, ginger, chilli)	as desired	0	
Spices, ground (e.g. paprika, chilli powder, curry powder)	as desired	0	
Spices, whole (e.g. cumin seeds, coriander seeds, caraway seeds)	as desired	0	
Spinach, canned, drained	as desired	0	
Spinach, frozen, steamed	as desired	0	
Spinach, raw	as desired	0	
Spinach, steamed	as desired	0	
Sponge cake	small slice	6	watch portion size
Spread, half fat, unsaturated	1 teaspoon	1	
Spread, half fat, unsaturated	scraping	0.5	some are mono-unsaturated
Spread, low-fat	scraping	0.5	
Spread, low-fat	1 teaspoon	1	
Spread, very low-fat, unsaturated	1 teaspoon	0.5	
Spring greens, steamed	as desired	0	
Spring onions, bulbs and tops, raw	as desired	0	
Squash, sugar-free	as desired	0	

Food	Portion Size	GiPs	Special Comments
Steak and kidney/Beef pie, individual, chilled/frozen, baked	1 pie	4.5	
Stock cube	small amounts	0	try low-sodium types
Strawberries	1 teacupful	0	keep to portion size if you want to have them GiP-free
Sugar	2 teaspoons	2.5	
Sultanas	2 handfuls	3	
Sushi	6 mini	2.5	
Swede, steamed	2 tablespoons	3	
Sweet potato, baked	1 small potato	3.5	
Sweet potato, boiled	1 small potato	3	
Sweet potato, steamed	1 small potato	3	
Sweet potato, steamed or microwaved	1 small potato	3	
Sweetcorn, baby, canned, drained	as desired	0	
Sweetcorn, baby, fresh and frozen, steamed	as desired	0	
Sweetcorn, kernels, canned, drained	3 tablespoons	2.5	choose canned veg in unsalted, unsweetened water
Sweetcorn, kernels, fresh, cooked	3 tablespoons	2.5	
Sweetcorn, on-the-cob, whole, steamed	1 cob	2	

T

Food	Portion Size	GiPs	Special Comments
Taco shells, baked	1 shell	7	
Tomato purée	as desired	0	
Tomatoes, canned, with juice	as desired	0	make a sauce with onion, garlic and herbs, add to pasta for a low-GiP meal
Tomatoes, cherry, raw	as desired	0	
Tomatoes, raw	as desired	0	
Tongue, ox, stewed	2 slices	2.5	
Tortillas, wheat	1 wrap	3	
Trout, steamed or grilled	1 fish	1.5	a source of healthy omega-3 fats

Food	Portion Size	GiPs	Special Comments
Tuna, canned in brine, drained	small can	1	half the calories of canned in oil
Turkey, roasted	2 slices	2	you get three times as much if you use wafer-thin turkey
Turnip, steamed	as desired	0	
Twix	1 mini Twix (21 g)	2.5	
Tzatziki	2 tablespoons	1	opt for lower-fat versions if available

V

Veal, cutlet, sautéed	1 cutlet	2.5	
Veal, fillet, roast	1 fillet	2.5	
Vine leaves, preserved in brine	as desired	0	
Vine leaves, stuffed with rice	8 medium vine leaves	3	
vinegar (rice, balsamic, malt, wine)	as desired	0	

W

Waffles	1 waffle	6.5	
Water, sparkling	as desired	0	
Water, still	as desired	0	
Water, sugar-free, flavoured	as desired	0	check no added sugar
Watercress, raw	as desired	0	
Worcestershire sauce	as desired	0	

Y

Yam, baked	size of a medium potato	1.5	
Yam, boiled	size of a medium potato	1.5	
Yam, steamed	size of a medium potato	1.5	
Yoghurt, diet	small pot	1	
Yoghurt, low-fat, natural	small pot	1	

PART FOUR

USEFUL INFO

FOOD AND MOOD DIARY

Food fills a physical hole, not an emotional need. When you become more aware of the underlying feeling that is causing you to overeat, you are more able to make some changes. Fill in this daily food journal to highlight the emotional need that causes you to have a snack attack. Remind yourself, 'What would

Time	Food Eaten & Quantity	Fruit & Veg	Points

TOTAL POINTS FOR THE DAY

have to happen, that is within my control, for this need to be met in a healthy and functional way?' Before you seek solace in that 'naughty but nice food', ask yourself whether this is taking you nearer to the 'new' you. If it isn't, choose again! (See pages 105-7 for more advice.) Recording what you eat will also help you to check if you are keeping to the GiP rules and, if not, what you might want to adjust next time.

Week Number. . . . .
Day/Date. . . . .
Working/non-working day . . . .

Emotions, e.g. tired, hungry, feeling low	Comments

HEALTHY FOOD TRACKER

This is your tracking system to see how well you're keeping in balance with the foods you eat and your lifestyle. The highlighted number are your targets. You might like to photocopy this page so you have a page for each day or week. Then you can see at a glance how well you're doing with keeping to healthy low-GI guidelines.

Which day is it?
Monday
Tuesday
Wednesday
Thursday
Friday
Saturday
Sunday

How are you doing?
Circle the number of portions (servings) you had today of the following:

Starchy carbs – such as bread, cereals, rice, pasta, potatoes (choose one serving at each meal).

1   2   **(3)**   4   5   6   7   8   9   10

Protein foods – such as meat, fish, eggs, cheese, nuts **(once a day only)**, beans (only one serving at each meal, max 3 per day).

1 2 ③ 4 5 6 7 8 9 10

Fruit and vegetables (at least 5 a day).

1 2 3 4 ⑤ 6 7 8 9 10

Sugary and fatty foods (such as biscuits, cakes, pastries, spreads, oils – keep 'em low).

1 2 3 4 5 6 7 8 9 10

Glasses of water (6–8 glasses: 1½–2 litres/3½–4½ pints a day).

1 2 3 4 5 6 7 ⑧ 9 10

Physical activity, such as brisk walk, running (two 10-minute bursts daily).

1 ② 3 4 5 6 7 8 9 10

Rank how positive or negative you are today (5 being the most positive and 1 being the most negative).

1 2 3 4 5

Rank your hunger today (1 means you're starving, 5 means you could do without your next snack).

1 2 3 4 5

Rank your energy today.

1 2 3 4 5

Rank your mood today.

1   2   3   4   5

Rank your self-esteem today.

1   2   3   4   5

How was breakfast?

❏ Had none.

❏ Grab and go, ditched the rules.

❏ Bent the rules but feel okay about it.

❏ Did just what I was supposed to do.

How was lunch?

❏ Had none.

❏ Grab and go, ditched the rules.

❏ Bent the rules but feel okay about it.

❏ Did just what I was supposed to do.

How was dinner?

❏ Had none.

❏ Grab and go, ditched the rules.

❏ Bent the rules but feel okay about it.

❏ Did just what I was supposed to do.

What about snacks?

❏ Had none.

❏ Grab and go, ditched the rules.

❏ Bent the rules but feel okay about it.

❏ Did just what I was supposed to do.

How do you rate yourself in general today?

1   2   3   4   5

What do you need right now to make this even better?

How can you achieve this?

What will you do?

ATTENTION SCIENCE ADDICTS!

RESEARCH, REFERENCES AND FURTHER READING

This section is for the real science addicts. It contains summaries of only some of the research on GI and weight loss as well as the published literature that we used as research for this book.

Summary of scientific research

1. Agus MSD, Swain JF, Larson CL, Eckert EA, Ludwig DS (2000). Dietary composition and physiologic adaptations to energy restriction. *American Journal of Clinical Nutrition* **71**:901–7.

Body weight set point has been suggested as an explanation for poor long-term results of conventional energy-restricted diets in the treatment of obesity. This study aimed to establish if dietary composition affects hormonal and metabolic adaptations to energy restriction. A randomised crossover design was used to compare the effects of a high-GI and a low-GI energy-restricted diet. Ten overweight males were studied for nine days on two separate occasions. The men freely selected foods for the first day and were then randomised to a high-GI energy-restricted diet (67 per cent CHO, 15 per cent protein, 18 per cent fat) or a low-GI energy-restricted diet (43 per cent CHO, 27 per cent protein, 30 per cent fat). The energy-restricted diets were consumed until day six. On days seven and eight the men remained on the high- or low-GI diets but were not energy restricted.

The men following the low-GI regime showed a greater level of serum leptin (a hormone that regulates appetite and energy expenditure), a higher resting energy expenditure, lower energy intake from snack foods and a preferential nitrogen balance (an indicator of protein breakdown) to the group who had followed the high-GI regime.

The authors conclude that physiological adaptations to energy restriction can be modified by dietary composition.

2. Bell SJ. Sears B (2003). Low-Glycaemic-load diets: Impact in obesity and chronic diseases. Critical Review in *Food Science and Nutrition* **43**(4): 357–77

This is a review of the data surrounding the public health messages of simple low-fat, high-carbohydrate diets and suggests we should be looking beyond Glycaemic Index (GI) and more closely at Glycaemic Load (GL). GL reflects the effect of the total day's carbohydrate on insulin secretion and hunger rather than that of individual foods. Foods such as carrots are shown to have a high GI but low GL, and therefore are recommended, while potatoes have a high GI and high GL and should be restricted.

A study at Harvard Medical School randomised 107 obese but otherwise healthy children into a low-GL diet group and a reduced-fat (25–30 per cent energy) diet group for four months. The low-GL group lost significantly more weight than the low-fat group with 17 per cent of subjects showing a reduction in BMI of $3kg/m^2$.

A 10-year multi-centre trial of healthy adults aged 18–39 concluded that a low-GL diet rich in dietary fibre was associated with reduced triglycerides, blood pressure, and LDL cholesterol, and increased HDL cholesterol. Similarly, the Nurses Health Study, which followed 75,521 women aged 38–63 with no history of CVD, concluded that high-fibre dietary GL was directly associated with CVD risk and recommended the classification of carbohydrates by GL.

Both the Nurses Health Study and the Health Professional Follow-up Study looking at 42,759 men showed up to a 40 per cent increased risk of developing diabetes in subjects following a high-GL diet to those consuming a low-GL diet. Both of these studies were not exclusively dietary interventions and therefore results may have been influenced by other factors.

Although the authors acknowledge that the current

data is mainly from short-term studies, **they suggest that public health messages should emphasise the need to incorporate low-GI, low-GL foods** into the diet and call for more long-term studies in the future.

3. Ludwig DS (2000). Dietary glycaemic index and obesity. *Journal of Nutrition* **130**:280S–83S.

This review examines the physiological effects of Glycaemic Index and argues for the need for controlled clinical trials of a low-Glycaemic Index (GI) diet in the treatment of obesity. **To date, at least 16 studies have examined the effects of GI on appetite and all but one have demonstrated an increase in satiety, delayed hunger return and reduced food intake following low-GI foods than following high-GI foods.** This study compared the effects of three meals of equal energy value comprising either high-GI, medium-GI or low-GI foods. Twelve teenage boys, otherwise healthy with at least 120 per cent ideal bodyweight, were evaluated on three separate occasions and randomly fed a test meal as a breakfast and again at lunch. The rapid absorption of glucose from the high-GI breakfast resulted in relatively high insulin and low glycagon concentrations. The same effects applied to test lunches, and subjects consumed significantly more energy after the high-GI lunch than either the medium- or low-GI meals.

While the authors accept there may not be a single optimal diet for the treatment of obesity, they suggest that diets designed to lower insulin response to ingested carbohydrate (for example, low GI) may improve access to stored metabolic fuels. Further, they may decrease hunger and promote weight loss. They go on to describe these diets as containing abundant fruits, vegetables and legumes with moderate amounts of protein and healthful fats and decreased refined carbohydrates and potatoes.

The authors remark on the similarity of the low-GI diet with the diet of human ancestors over the last several hundred years.

4. Brand-Miller JC, Holt SHA, Pawlak DB, McMillan J (2002). Glycaemic index and obesity. *American Journal of Clinical Nutrition* 76:281S–285S.

Although weight loss can be achieved by any means of energy restriction, current dietary guidelines have not prevented weight regain or population-level increases in obesity and overweight. Many high-carbohydrate, low-fat diets may be counterproductive to weight control because they markedly increase postprandial hyperglycaemia and hyperinsulinaemia. Many high-carbohydrate foods common to Western diets produce a high glycaemic response, promoting postprandial carbohydrate oxidation at the expense of fat oxidation, which may promote body-fat increases. In contrast, diets based on low-fat foods that produce a low glycaemic response may enhance weight control because they promote satiety, minimise postprandial insulin secretion, and maintain insulin sensitivity.

This hypothesis is supported by several intervention studies in humans in which energy-restricted diets based on low-GI foods produced greater weight loss than equivalent diets based on high-GI foods. Long-term studies in animal models have also shown that diets based on high-GI starches promote weight gain, visceral adiposity, and higher concentrations of fat-metabolising enzymes than do low-GI starch-controlled diets of equivalent energy value.

In an eight-week study of 12 healthy pregnant women, a high-GI diet was associated with greater weight at term than was a nutrient-balanced, low-GI diet. In a study of diet and complications of nearly 3,000 subjects with type 1 diabetes, the GI of the overall diet was an independent predictor of waist circumference in men.

The authors conclude that the findings of this review provide scientific rationale to justify randomised, controlled, multi-centre intervention studies comparing the effects of conventional and low-GI diets on weight control.

5. McManus K, Antinoro L, Sacks F (2001). A randomised controlled trial of a moderate-fat low-energy diet with a low-fat, low-energy diet for weight loss in overweight adults. *International Journal of Obesity,* **25**, 5: 1503–1511.

Nutrition experts studied 101 overweight men and

women, who followed either a moderate-fat diet (35 per cent energy from fat), or a standard low-fat diet (20 per cent energy from fat). Both groups ate the same total calories (women: 1200 kcal; men: 1500 kcal). The moderate-fat diet encouraged inclusion of good sources of monounsaturated fats such as peanuts, peanut butter, olive oil, rapeseed oil, avocados and other nuts, all foods typically forbidden on standard low-fat diets. Saturated-fat intake was kept low. Subjects could consume peanut butter at breakfast and 25 g/1 oz nut snacks each afternoon on the 1200 kcal diet.

Results showed a greater participation rate for those on the moderate-fat diet that included nuts, with over half sticking to the diet, compared to only one in five sticking to the low-fat diet over the 18-month study period. Both groups lost an average of 5 kg/11 lb in the first year, although it is the longer-term results that really distinguish the diets. Those following the moderate-fat diet were able to keep off a significant amount of their lost weight, whereas the low-fat group had regained some of their initial weight loss at 18 months. Those on the moderate-fat diet had still managed to keep off a significant amount of weight 2½ years after the start of the study. **After 18 months the group which ate 25 g nuts as part of a healthy diet had reduced their waist size by 6.9 cm/2¾ in, whereas the other group had in fact increased theirs by 2.6 cm/1 in.**

6. Matthias B, Schulze DRPH, Frank B Hu MD (2004). Dietary approaches to prevent the metabolic syndrome. Quality versus quantity of carbohydrates. *Diabetes Care*, **27**:2.

Prevailing dietary guidelines continue to recommend very high intakes of grain products without a clear distinction between whole and refined grains*. Many popular diets that focus on weight loss, on the other hand, have jumped on the low-carbohydrate bandwagon, prohibiting virtually all carbohydrates, especially in the initial phase of the diet. Both approaches are incompatible with current scientific evidence and can have long-term adverse health implications. **With the growing epidemic of obesity and the metabolic syndrome, reduction in the consumption of refined carbohydrates and sugar, replaced by minimally processed wholegrain products and healthy sources of fats and protein, should become a major public health priority, together with regular physical activity and weight maintenance.**

References and further reading

Foster-Powell K, Holt SHA, Brand-Miller JC (2002). International table of glycemic index and glycemic load values (2002). *American Journal of Clinical Nutrition* **76**:266S–273S.

* US Department of Agriculture, US Department of Heath and Human Services: *Nutrition and Your Health: Dietary Guidelines for Americans*. Washington, DC, US Government Printing Office, 2000.

Jenkins DJA, Kendall CWC, Augustin LSA et al. (2002). Glycemic index: overview of implications in health and disease. *American Journal of Clinical Nutrition* **76**:266S–273S.

Ludwig DS, Majzoub JA, Al-Zahrani A, Dallal GE, Blanco I, Roberts SB (1999). High glycemic index foods, overeating, and obesity. *Pediatrics* 103(3).

Food and Agriculture Organisation/World Health Organisation. Carbohydrates in Human Nutrition. Report of a Joint FAO/WHO Expert Consultation. Rome, 14–18 April 1997. *FAO Food and Nutrition Paper* 66, 1998.

Jiang R, Manson JE, Stampfer MJ, Liu S, Willett WC, Hu FB (2002). A prospective study of nut consumption and risk of type 2 diabetes in women. *Journal of the American Medical Association* **288**: 2554–2560.

The New Glucose Revolution (formerly *The GI Factor*), by Dr Anthony Leeds, Prof. Jennie Brand Miller, Kaye Foster-Powell and Dr Stephen Colagiuri. Published by Hodder and Stoughton (2003).

ABOUT THE AUTHORS

Azmina Govindji BSc RD is a consultant nutritionist and registered dietitian, broadcaster, best-selling author and Master NLP Practitioner.

She started her early career as a clinical dietitian in several hospitals (gaining direct experience with patients). She then spent eight years as the National Consultant on Diet and Diabetes when she was Chief Dietitian to Diabetes UK. This experience makes her particularly qualified to write this book, as GI is a concept that has been used in diabetes for years. She now runs her own practice providing dietetic consultancy to the food industry, healthcare professionals, the media, and national organisations such as the British Heart Foundation and Diabetes Research and Wellness Foundation. She is currently Chairperson of the British Dietetic Association (BDA) PR Committee and a member of the BDA Executive Council.

In 2002 Azmina won the Ismaili Community National Award for Excellence for outstanding professional achievement, as judged by Professor Kenneth Calman, former chief medical officer to the government.

A regular contributor to numerous magazines, she also appears on TV and radio, and is frequently quoted in the national press as spokesperson for the British Dietetic Association. Azmina has worked on two diabetes education videos with *GMTV*'s Dr Hilary Jones and is author of 10 books, including **Healthy Eating for Diabetes** with Anthony Worrall Thompson, and **Think Well to Be Well** with Nina Puddefoot. Her website is www.azminagovindji.com

Nina Puddefoot is a Master Practitioner and Certified NLP Trainer and development life coach. She works with leading-edge and creative models of thinking within multinational organisations and industries as well as individuals worldwide.

She is an author and a regular presenter of public programmes, talks and workshops and has appeared as a guest speaker on *The Aurora*.

Nina has been featured in a series of programmes about business and health for cable television and regularly makes contributions to radio, newspapers and magazines, including *The Daily Mail*, *New Woman* and *Family Circle*.

She is renowned for her ability to quickly establish relationships with sensitivity and humour and for enriching and inspiring the lives of others through her support for individuals' empowerment and passion.

FURTHER INFORMATION AND SUPPORT

Visit Az and Nina on www.gipointdiet.com and www.thinkwelltobewell.com

www.gipointdiet.com is a supportive site for anyone wanting to get into GI-eating by using the Gi Point Diet and motivational strategies. If you've already bought the book and need a quick inspirational 'top-up', or some new menu ideas, this is worth a visit. For the uninitiated, www.gipointdiet.com will simply whet your appetite.

The *Think Well to Be Well* website offers golden nuggets of information and inspires you to check and challenge your thinking, approach and attitudes to food choices and many aspects of life. It offers willpower boosters, slimming tips, and a host of information on diet and diabetes.

Books

Think Well to Be Well by Azmina Govindji and Nina Puddefoot. Published by Diabetes Research &

Wellness Foundation (2002).

Rosie's Armchair Exercises by Rosita Evans. Published by Discovery Books, 29 Hacketts Lane, Woking, GU22 8PP. Tel: 01932 400800.

Leaflets on *Healthy Eating in Diabetes* (incorporating low-GI foods) for South Asian, Arabic and Western food ideas. Available from:

Sunita Wallia

Community Dietitian

Greater Glasgow Primary Care NHS Trust

120 William St Clinic

Glasgow G3 8UR

Tel: 0141 314 6234

Organisations

Registered dietitians hold the only legally recognisable graduate qualification in nutrition and dietetics. If you would like to visit a dietitian, contact:

British Dietetic Association

5th Floor, Charles House

148/9 Great Charles Street

Queensway

Birmingham B3 3HT

Tel: 0121 200 8080

Diabetes Research and Wellness Foundation (DRWF)

The DRWF is a charity working to help people with

diabetes and related illnesses.
Diabetes Research and Wellness Foundation
Northney Marina
Hayling Island
Hants
PO11 0NH
Tel: 023 9263 7808

Diabetes UK
10 Parkway
London NW1 7AA
Tel: 020 7424 1000

Websites

The British Dietetic Association sites include:
www.bda.uk.com
www.weightwisebda.uk.com

For diabetes-specific sites, visit:
www.diabeteswellnessnet.org.uk
www.diabetes.org.uk

Also visit: www.azminagovindji.com

INDEX

Note: 'GiP' refers to Gi Point, and 'GI' refers to Glycaemic Index